Praise for the *Intelligent Patient Guide* series

The guide to breast cancer walks you through each step of your diagnosis, treatment and prognosis...with explanations that are easily understood. It brought everything together, making it so clear.

— J. McIntosh, Patient

One of the best explanations of breast cancer risk I've seen in print...dispels the 'panic' of the '1 in 9' statistics... It's lovely to see in print many of the teachings we use on a daily basis.

— Barbara Warren, RN,
Director of Nursing,
CancerCare Manitoba

As a patient advocate and breast cancer survivor, I lend and use my copy of the Intelligent Patient Guide often. The book helps equip patients to better understand the need to take charge in the design of their own survival.

— B. Cameron

It was so informative. I felt so secure knowing what was going to happen with every step.

— D. Powell, Patient

A tremendous tool that I make available to all my patients.

— Dr. J. Caines, Halifax, Nova Scotia

I found the Intelligent Patient Guide an excellent tool during my recent surgery and treatments. It gave me a sense of being an active participant on the road to recovery.

— S. Moorhouse, RN, Patient

Intelligent Patient Guide To

Breast Cancer

Other books in the *Intelligent Patient Guide*
series include:

The Intelligent Patient Guide to Prostate Cancer, 3rd edition
by S. Larry Goldenberg, MD, Ian M. Thompson, MD
ISBN 0-9696125-5-9

The Intelligent Patient Guide to Colorectal Cancer, 2nd edition
by Michael E. Pezim, MD, David Owen, MB
ISBN 0-9696125-7-5

Intelligent Patient Guide To

Breast Cancer

*All you need to know to take
an active part in your treatment*

Ivo Olivotto, MD
Karen Gelmon, MD
David McCready, MD
Kathleen Pritchard, MD
Urve Kuusk, MD

edited by
Cheryl Edwards, MA

INTELLIGENT
PATIENT GUIDE

Fourth edition, Vancouver, 2006

While the authors have made every effort to ensure that the material contained herein is accurate at time of publication, new discoveries or changes in treatment practices may ultimately invalidate some of the information presented here.

Intelligent Patient Guide Ltd.
Suite 30, 3195 Granville Street
Vancouver, British Columbia V6H 3K2
Canada
e-mail: info@ipguide.com
fax: 604-876-9334

Fifth printing, 2009

Library and Archives Canada Cataloguing in Publication

The intelligent patient guide to breast cancer / Ivo Olivotto ... [et al.] ; edited by Cheryl Edwards ; illustrated by Jane Rowlands.—4th ed.

(Intelligent patient guide)
Includes index.
Previous eds. written by Ivo Olivotto, Karen Gelmon, Urve Kuusk.
ISBN 0-9696125-8-3
ISBN 978-0-9696125-8-2

1. Breast—Cancer—Popular works. I. Olivotto, Ivo, 1956-
II. Edwards Cheryl III. Series.

RC280.B8I57 2006   616.99'449   C2005-907475-2

Cover design by MURPHYWOODS Creative & Design, Vancouver
Graphic Production by Angela G. Atkins, North Vancouver
Printed in Canada

Distributed by
Gordon Soules Book Publishers Ltd.
1359 Ambleside Lane,
West Vancouver, BC, Canada V7T 2Y9
E-mail: books@gordonsoules.com
604-922-6588 Fax: 604-688-5442

This book is dedicated to the thousands of women who have lived and are living with breast cancer and who, through their stories and their strength, have taught us so much.

Authors

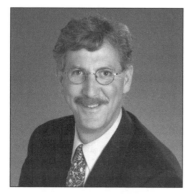

Ivo Olivotto, MD

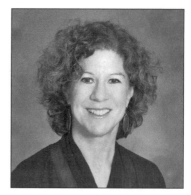

Karen Gelmon, MD

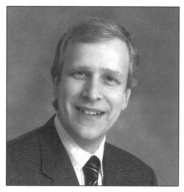

David McCready, MD

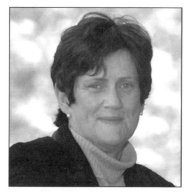

Kathleen Pritchard, MD

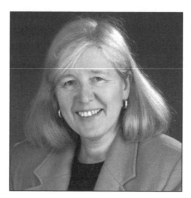

Urve Kuusk, MD

Authors

Ivo Olivotto, MD, FRCPC
Head
Breast Cancer Outcomes Unit
BC Cancer Agency;
Professor
Division of Radiation Oncology
University of British Columbia

David McCready, MD, MSc,
FRCSC, FACS
Gattuso Chair in Breast Surgical
    Oncology
Department of Surgical Oncology
Princess Margaret Hospital
Mt Sinai Hospital
Professor of Surgery
University of Toronto

Urve Kuusk, MD, FRCPC
Clinical Associate Professor
Division of General Surgery
University of British Columbia

Karen Gelmon, MD, FRCPC
Clinical Head
Section of Investigational New
    Drugs
Chair, Breast Tumor Group
BC Cancer Agency;
Clinical Professor
Division of Medical Oncology
University of British Columbia

Kathleen Pritchard, MD, FRCPC
Head
Clinical Trials and Epidemiology
Chair, Breast Cancer Site Group
Toronto Sunnybrook Regional
    Cancer Center;
Professor
Department of Medicine
University of Toronto

Editor
Cheryl Edwards, MA

Illustrator
Jane Rowlands

Coordinator
Nicola Sutton, MBA

Series Medical Director
Michael E. Pezim, MD, FRCSC

Contributing Authors

Judith Caldwell
Founder, Canadian Breast Cancer
    Foundation
British Columbia/Yukon Chapter

Paula Gordon, MD, FRCPC
Clinical Associate Professor
    Department of Radiology
University of British Columbia

Susan Harris, PT, PhD
Professor, School of Rehabilitation
    Sciences
University of British Columbia

Charmaine Kim-Sing, MD,
FRCPC
Medical Leader, Hereditary
    Cancer Program
BC Cancer Agency and University
    of British Columbia

Michael Shew, BSc, MBA
Patient Education Group Member
BC Cancer Agency

Lis Smith, CCH
Clinical Hypnotherapist

Cheri Van Patten, MSc, RDN
Registered Dietician-Nutritionist
BC Cancer Agency

Richard Warren, MD, FRCSC
Head, Division of Plastic Surgery
University of British Columbia

The authors of this book and the management of Intelligent Patient Guide Ltd., mourn the untimely death of Dr. Patty Clugston on March 1, 2005. Patty was the co-founder of the British Columbia Breast Reconstruction Program and was a tireless advocate for improved care for women with breast cancer. Her loss will be keenly felt by both her patients and colleagues.

Why read this book?

AFTER YOUR DOCTOR SAYS the words 'breast cancer' you may be in a state of shock. Despite this, you will be expected to make a series of major decisions, often in a hurry. 'Should I have a mastectomy? Should I have radiation? Chemotherapy? Tamoxifen?' The choices seem so complicated. Women often end up wondering, 'Should I just leave the decisions up to my doctors and do whatever they suggest?'

We believe not. Time and again we have seen that the patient who takes an active part in making the decisions that affect the course of her treatment is better able to cope than the patient who relegates all control to her doctors. While we are not advocating that you make choices independently of the recommendations of your doctor, we encourage you to become one of the decision-makers.

Since first publishing this book in 1995 and updating it in 1998 and in 2001, we have been gratified to hear from many women who have found the information useful. It has helped them understand the disease, ask doctors the questions they needed to ask, and make the decisions they needed to make about their treatment.

Progress is always being made, and as soon as a book is written there may be aspects of care that change or come into question. As much as we regret these discrepancies, we applaud any progress that will improve the care of women with breast cancer.

It is important to note that the statistics we have quoted about risks and prognosis refer to general or 'average' situations. Special additional circumstances may modify your individual risk and need to be discussed with your doctor.

We hope this book can help you move through the fear, to a place of hope and strength and the promise of life ahead—in spite of breast cancer.

Ivo Olivotto, MD
Karen Gelmon, MD
David McCready, MD
Kathleen Pritchard, MD
Urve Kuusk, MD

Table of contents

PART ONE | **Breast Cancer:
What is it and
how is it detected?**

What is breast cancer?

CHAPTER ONE

What is cancer?

TO UNDERSTAND CANCER, it is important to learn about normal growth in the body.

How does the body grow and maintain itself?

The body is made up of billions of tiny cells. During normal growth, a cell becomes larger, and then divides into two 'daughter' cells (Figure 1). After a period of time, each of these cells divides again. Our bodies experience a lot of wear and tear so old or worn out cells constantly need to be replaced. Normally this happens in an orderly, systematic way because each cell carries genetic instructions that regulate how fast the cell should divide and grow and when the cell should die. A balance between cells growing and dying keeps our bodies functioning normally.

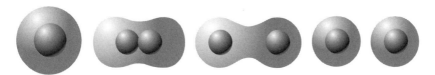

Figure 1: Normal cell division. A cell grows a bit larger and then divides into two cells.

When cell growth goes out of control

Benign growths

Sometimes cells disregard the normal balance between cell growth and death. As a result, a small, harmless lump of cells called a 'benign' growth may form. A benign growth can occur in any part of the body.

Malignant growths

In other cases, cells may grow into a large mass or spread to other areas of the body. Cells that have this aggressive behavior are called 'malignant.' More commonly, a mass of such cells is called a 'cancer'. When clumps of these cells spread to other parts of the body, they are called 'metastases'. Eventually, a cancer that continues to grow can overwhelm and destroy the part of the body or organ where it is located.

Cancer cells also have the ability to stimulate the development of blood vessels to increase their own blood supply and enhance their growth. This is called 'angiogenesis'. Sometimes, a cancer may outgrow its oxygen and nutrient supply, and when this happens, a part of the cancer may suddenly die. The death of a group of cells within a cancer is known as 'necrosis'.

Cancer cells have the ability to spread

Unlike cancer cells, normal cells remain in the area of the body where they belong, never spreading to other parts. However, cancer cells can spread through the body (metastasize) in several ways (Figure 2). These include: direct invasion and destruction of the organ of origin, or spread through the lymphatic system and/or blood stream to distant organs such as the lungs, liver or bones.

When a cancer spreads, it retains the properties of the original cancer. This means that a breast cancer that has spread to the bones is still a breast cancer. Under the microscope it still looks like breast cancer and looks different than a cancer that started in the bone. When a breast cancer has spread it continues to behave like a breast cancer, not a cancer from the organ to which it has spread, for instance the lung or bone.

The original cancer in the breast is called the 'primary' cancer. A cancer that has spread to another site is called a 'secondary' or 'metastatic' cancer.

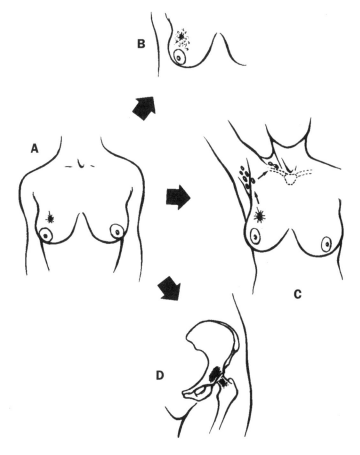

Figure 2: How breast cancer spreads. A cancer (A) grows and spreads by direct local invasion (B) of the breast itself or (C) through the lymphatic system to lymph nodes or (D) through the blood stream to distant organs such as the bones, lungs, liver or brain.

Breast cancer does not develop overnight

It can take years of cells dividing before a normal cell becomes a cancerous cell. The cell first undergoes very small changes which may not be detectable or may appear slightly abnormal or atypical under a microscope. The cell may also begin to divide, grow more quickly and accumulate in excessive numbers (hyperplasia). Then, over the years, these cells continue to change, appear more abnormal looking and finally become cancerous (Figure 3).

Initially the cancer cells are confined within the milk ducts (*in situ* cancers), but with time, the cells develop the ability to spread beyond the ducts and into the blood and lymphatic system (an *invasive* cancer).

Present technology cannot detect one or even a few cancer cells. It is only possible to detect small lumps of cancer cells. By the time a cancer is detected as a 1 cm lump, it contains about one billion cells and has been growing for two to eight years.

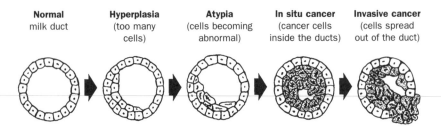

| **Normal**
milk duct | **Hyperplasia**
(too many
cells) | **Atypia**
(cells becoming
abnormal) | **In situ cancer**
(cancer cells
inside the ducts) | **Invasive cancer**
(cells spread
out of the duct) |

Figure 3: Breast cancer does not develop overnight. Cells gradually become more abnormal-looking or atypical (see text). Eventually, the cells are recognized as being sufficiently abnormal to be called cancer cells. They are initially inside the milk ducts (in situ cancer) and later develop into invasive breast cancer.

CHAPTER TWO

How common is breast cancer?

BREAST CANCER IS THE MOST COMMON TYPE of cancer in women. In 2006 there will be about 23,000 new cases diagnosed in Canada leading to over 5,000 deaths (and approximately ten times that number in the USA). Breast cancer accounts for 4% of all deaths of women in North America each year and the loss of thousands of productive years of life.

'One in nine' is misleading

One often hears that 'one in nine' women will get breast cancer. The trouble with this figure is that it can be misleading because the risk of breast cancer increases with age. The ratio 'one in nine' refers to the chance that a woman will develop breast cancer if she lives to the age of 90. Women over 70, for example, are four times more likely to get breast cancer than 40 years olds. Since many women die of other causes before the age of 90, they don't actually reach the age group at highest risk.

Recent changes in the incidence of breast cancer

The number of new cases diagnosed each year per 100,000 women is called the 'incidence'. Since the 1940s, there has been a slow but steady increase in the number of new cases of breast cancer diagnosed each year in North America. This increase has been attributed to changes in nutrition, such as consumption of more calories, and changes in reproductive patterns. Today, women start menstruating several years earlier, delay having babies and have fewer children. These factors tend to increase exposure of the maturing breast to estrogens and have been linked to the higher rates of breast cancer.

In addition, there was a definite increase in the incidence of breast cancer (more than 1% per year) reported in the mid-1980s. That was largely due to the increased use of screening mammograms which can detect some cancers two to five years before a lump can be felt by the woman or her doctor. As most women had at least one mammogram during the 1980s and 1990s, the sudden wave of earlier detected cancers passed, and the incidence rates dropped back to the background rate prior to the screening era.

You can estimate your own risk

Rather than considering a lifetime risk to age 90, a more useful question is: 'What is my risk, given my current age?'

Table 1 shows the average risk each year of developing breast cancer for typical North American women at specific ages. Using Table 1, based on her current age, the 'average' woman can estimate her risk of developing breast cancer over the next year. The risk over the next decade is 10 times the annual risk. For example, if you are 42, your annual risk is slightly higher than that of the 40-year-old listed in Table 1, say 1/1,000 per year. Over the next decade your risk would be 10 x 1/1,000 = 1/100 or approximately 1% over the next ten years. This risk is much easier to live with than one in nine.

Table 1 Annual (not lifetime) risk of developing breast cancer	
At age	**Risk**
30 years	1 in 6,000 per year
40 years	1 in 1,200 per year
50 years	1 in 550 per year
60 years	1 in 400 per year
70 years	1 in 300 per year
80 years	1 in 250 per year

Table 2 shows not the annual risk, but the lifetime risk up to certain ages. As you can see from Table 2, even a woman who is 75 years old does not yet have a 'one in nine' chance of developing breast cancer. More specific, individualized risk estimates can be determined by considering additional factors that are associated with a higher risk of developing breast cancer, and then multiplying the 'average' risk at a certain age by the risk factor. A web-based model to calculate the risk of developing breast cancer for women without a previous breast cancer can be found at: http:/brca.nci.nih.gov/brc/. Chapter 3 discusses some of the causes of breast cancer and ranks them according to their importance.

Table 2 **Chance of developing breast cancer by a given age**	
Age	**Lifetime risk**
by 25 years	less than 1 in 1,000
by 50 years	1 in 63
by 75 years	1 in 15
by 90 years	1 in 9

CHAPTER THREE

What causes breast cancer?

Why me?

'WHY DID I GET BREAST CANCER?' This is a question that doctors can almost never answer with any accuracy. However, it is not your 'fault' or 'punishment' for something you did or did not do, and it is not something you subconsciously 'needed.' Breast cancer is not something to be ashamed of.

There has been a lot of controversy over the years about the possible causes of breast cancer: diet, hormones, genetic make-up or substances in the environment. Today we realize that there is no single factor that causes breast cancer, but that it is a combination of things, some more important than others.

What is a risk factor?

A 'risk factor' refers to something that increases your chances of getting a disease, in this case, breast cancer. A strong risk factor greatly increases the chances, while a weak risk factor just slightly increases your chances. For example, in the case of lung cancer, smoking is a very strong risk factor since a smoker is far more likely to get lung cancer than a non-smoker.

With breast cancer there are several known risk factors, ranging from strong to weak (see Table 3).

Table 3 **Risk factors associated with the development of breast cancer**		
Strong (Risk greater than 4 x normal)	**Moderate** (Risk between 2–4 x normal)	**Weak** (Risk between 1–2 x normal)
Female sex	Over 30 years old at birth of first child	First menses before the age of 12 years
Advancing age		Menopause after the age of 54 years
Previous breast cancer (especially lobular carcinoma)	Past breast biopsy: any sign of cell abnormality or hyperplasia	Family history of breast cancer if the affected relatives were all older or postmenopausal
Family history of breast cancer if premenopausal or in both breasts	Postmenopausal obesity	
	Diet	Prolonged postmenopausal hormone use
Past breast biopsy showing severely abnormal cells and hyperplasia		Moderate to heavy alcohol consumption
		Certain ethnic origins

A 'strong' risk factor is defined as something that increases the chance of getting breast cancer by more than four times compared to someone without this risk factor. 'Moderate' means an increase of two to four times the risk, and 'weak' means less than two times the risk.

Strong risk factors

Increasing age is a strong risk factor for developing breast cancer. Women who are 50 years old have double the risk of women who are 40, and the risk doubles again by the age of 70 years (see Table 1). For three-quarters of the women who get breast cancer, age is the only identifiable risk factor. The remaining 25% of women with breast cancer have a combination of other risk factors.

Previous history of breast cancer

Most women who get one breast cancer do not get another. However, every year about one in every 200 women with a first breast cancer will develop another cancer in the opposite breast. Women with the lobular type of breast cancer (Chapter 14) have a higher chance, about 1% per year, of getting cancer in the opposite breast. Taking a anticancer hormone (a drug) like tamoxifen or an aromatase inhibitor (Arimidex®, Femara®, or Aromasin®—see Chapter 30) reduces the chance of developing a second cancer. However, it is still important to keep the second breast under surveillance with regular self and physician examinations and a yearly mammogram (breast x-ray).

Family history of breast cancer

A family history of breast cancer in a close relative such as your mother, sister or daughter contributes to your risk. However, breast cancer in only one distant relative such as an aunt or grandmother has little or no impact on your risk. A history of breast cancer in a pre-menopausal close relative, breast cancer in more than one close relative, or cancer in both breasts of a close relative confers a four to six times higher risk of developing breast cancer compared to a woman of the same age who does not have relatives with breast cancer.

There are rare families in which three or more generations have several relatives with breast cancer. In some of these families the disease may be passed on by a specific genetic mutation. For example, families with the BRCA1 or BRCA2 gene inherit a tendency to develop both breast and ovarian cancer. Women who inherit such a mutation have a lifetime risk of developing breast cancer as high as 85%. Many of these families are characterized by breast cancer developing before the age of 50. The disease may appear five to ten years earlier with each generation (see Chapter 41).

Moderate risk factors

Later pregnancy

The delivery of a first child before the age of 20 causes hormonal changes in the breast tissue which provide modest protection against breast cancer. Delaying the first child until after the age of 30 or having no full-term pregnancies increases the risk two to four times. Breastfeeding may decrease the chance of getting breast cancer by a small amount. In cultures where women breast feed each child for three or four years, this effect may be much greater.

Previous breast biopsy showing abnormal cells (atypia) or excessive accumulation of cells (hyperplasia)

As described in Chapter 1, a normal cell becomes a cancer cell through a series of changes in which the cells begin to divide and accumulate in excessive numbers (hyperplasia), become abnormal (atypical) and finally develop into cancer cells. If hyperplasia is seen in tissue removed during a breast biopsy, especially with atypical cells, the woman has a two to four times greater chance of developing breast cancer compared to a woman without these changes. If there is severe atypia and hyperplasia, especially in a woman who also has a family history of breast cancer, an eight-fold increased risk can be expected.

Weak risk factors

Generally, women who use oral contraceptives do not increase their risk of breast cancer. Some studies suggest that there is a modestly higher risk among women who, when they were young, took the older, high-dose estrogen type of pill for more than seven to ten years continuously. Modern oral contraceptive pills have a lower estrogen content, and do not increase the risk of developing breast cancer.

The onset of menstrual periods before the age of 12 years and cessation of menstruation after the age of 54 years weakly increase the risk of breast cancer.

Postmenopausal estrogen

The risk associated with postmenopausal hormone use ('hormone replacement therapy') is more controversial. Overall, women who have at some point used postmenopausal estrogens, alone or in combination with progesterone, have a modestly higher chance of developing breast cancer as compared with women who have never used these medications. Women who have taken post-menopausal hormones for longer than seven to 15 years have an approximately 1.5-fold increased risk compared to the risk among non-users. This modestly higher breast cancer risk has to be considered in context with the potentially beneficial effects of these medications, including, among other things, a lower risk of bone fractures and relief of hot flashes, vaginal dryness and mood swings which may accompany menopause.

Diet and body weight

There has been extensive research into the role of diet in the formation of breast cancer. Some authorities believe that up to 30% of breast cancers may be attributable to dietary influences.

Studies of populations which move from an area of low breast cancer risk (e.g. Japan) to an area of high risk (e.g. North America) show that within one to two generations the migrant population adopts the risk level of the new country. This is thought to be due to changes of diet and life-style which the children and grandchildren of the immigrants adopt.

It is not clear which dietary factors are important in causing breast cancer but the principal culprit is thought to be dietary fat. Furthermore, it is not known which type of dietary fat may be the culprit: saturated or unsaturated, fat of vegetable or animal origin, or whether the effect is simply related to eating too many calories.

Obesity and an increase in body mass index (BMI) appear to be associated with an increase in breast cancer risk in the post menopausal years. This may relate to the hormonal changes that occur in the body with obesity including changes in how the body responds to insulin. The impact of body weight on the risk of developing breast cancer however is confusing as women who are markedly underweight in the premenopausal years, also experience an increased risk of breast cancer.

Moderate to heavy alcohol consumption (more than three drinks or six glasses of wine per week) has been associated with a weak increase in the risk of developing breast cancer. However, it remains reasonable to have an occasional drink or glass of wine.

Environmental factors

Radiation from x-rays is a common concern. Even at low doses, the use of repeated x-rays in younger women (less than 20 years old) has been associated with an increased risk of breast cancer. The usual dose of radiation from a mammogram (x-ray of the breast) is very small. Since routine mammograms tend to be used in women older than 40 years and since older women tend to be more resistant to the effects of radiation than younger women, the chance that a mammogram will cause a breast cancer is very low. Most authorities estimate that the small risk of causing a breast cancer is considerably less than the benefit that a mammogram may offer by revealing breast cancer earlier. (Chapter 6).

Chemical carcinogens are everywhere in our environment, but no specific chemical or substance has been identified as specifically causing a greater number of breast cancers. Although there has been concern about organochlorines found in pesticides, so far no direct association has been confirmed between the use of pesticides and incidence of breast cancer.

Smoking does not appear to significantly increase or decrease the risk of developing breast cancer except in one study suggesting that smoking within five years of a woman's first period increased the risk of breast cancer.

Race: little if any effect on risk

Historically, in the USA, blacks have had a lower incidence of breast cancer than whites, but unfortunately the survival rate for blacks is lower than the survival rate for whites. This has been attributed to differences in access to medical care rather than biological differences between races. In Canada, the age-adjusted risk among First Nations women seems to be lower than among caucasians.

Ethnic groups who migrate to North America from areas of low risk (e.g. Japan and Southeast Asia) adopt the higher risk of the 'average' woman in North America within one to two generations. This strongly suggests that the influences of race and ethnic background have little, if any role compared to diet, life-style or other environmental factors.

CHAPTER FOUR

Prevention—Is it possible?

Risk factors we cannot change

IT IS FRUSTRATING THAT THE MAJOR known risk factors for developing breast cancer cannot be changed, such as female sex, advancing age, family or previous personal history of breast cancer and the age at which menstrual periods begin (see Chapter 3). Getting pregnant at a very young age may have a weak protective effect but there are many reasons why delaying pregnancy may be more important.

Risk and health factors that we can change

Life-style factors

Life-style changes have been shown to reduce the chance of developing heart attacks, strokes and some cancers. Some studies indicate that regular exercise (four hours or more per week) or heavy manual labor at work can reduce the chance of getting breast cancer. It is not known why this happens, whether it is due to changes in hormone levels which occur with vigorous exercise, athletes' eating habits or perhaps the different amounts of body fat carried by active and inactive women. This area requires further study, but several hours per week of regular exercise is to be encouraged.

Stress has many different meanings and personal interpretations but usually involves a sense of loss of control or low self-esteem.

Making positive changes to reduce your personal level of stress can have substantial health benefits but may not affect cancer risk.

Diet

Diet is clearly an important factor in the development of breast cancer and is something which you can change. However, there is no specific diet that can guarantee that breast cancer will not develop. There is no simple remedy to prevent breast cancer in spite of what one reads on the newsstands. A healthy diet would consist of reducing your total amount of calories eaten and reducing the proportion of calories taken as fat to between 20% and 30% of your total calorie intake. This can be achieved by trimming the visible fat from meat, using leaner cuts, limiting pastries and chocolate, avoiding sauces rich in fat or cream, and substituting low fat milk products (skim or 1%) for the higher fat alternatives. Increasing the amount of green and yellow vegetables, which contain vitamin A, and the fiber content of the diet is to be encouraged (see Chapter 35). It is generally felt that drinking less alcohol may be beneficial, but it is not known how much is safe or what is too much.

Hormones

Moderate use of oral contraceptives and postmenopausal estrogens may have more advantages with respect to general health than disadvantages in terms of breast cancer risk. However, limiting postmenopausal estrogen use to less than 10 years where feasible may help reduce the chance of getting breast cancer.

Tamoxifen, an 'anti-estrogen' drug, is used for some types of breast cancer (see Chapter 30). A large North American study tested the value of tamoxifen as a method of preventing breast cancer. Over 13,000 women who had five times higher than the normal risk of developing breast cancer volunteered for this study. Tamoxifen was shown to reduce the chance of developing breast cancer and hip fractures, but increased the chance of developing blood clots in the legs and lungs and the chance of getting cancer of the endometrium (uterus). Tamoxifen is not recommended as prevention for all women. However, for a woman at very high risk of developing breast cancer (those at more than five times the average risk) taking tamoxifen for five years may have more benefits than risks. Women should discuss their individual risk of breast cancer and the likelihood of complications from tamoxifen with their doctors. A breast cancer risk assessment tool can be found at http://hcca.nci.nih.gov/brc.

Raloxifene, another anti-estrogen used for osteoporosis is being studied as a breast cancer prevention agent. Raloxifene also causes hot flashes and an increased risk of phlebitis, but should have a lower risk of endometrial cancer. Aromatase inhibitors such as Arimidex and Aromasin are also being studied as prevention drugs for postmenopausal women.

Surgical prevention

Rarely, a family may have breast cancer in three or more generations with several members of each generation affected. Much research is now aimed at identifying specific genes that will indicate which women in these families have an extremely high risk of developing breast cancer. Two such genes, called 'BRCA1' and 'BRCA2' were discovered in 1994. Women who have inherited mutations in the BRCA1 gene have a 50% to 85% chance of developing breast cancer and a 45% chance of developing ovarian cancer. Women with BRCA2 mutations have a high risk of breast cancer, as do men in the family, but a lower, yet still significant, risk of ovarian cancer. (Chapter 41 discusses family risks and genetic testing in more detail.)

Surgical prevention (removal of both breasts) is a drastic measure that should be considered only by women with a very high risk (50% or higher) of getting breast cancer who have participated in counseling and weighed the alternatives carefully. This procedure is called 'prophylactic mastectomy.' If both breasts are to be removed as a preventive measure, then the nipples and all the underlying breast tissue should be removed. It is not necessary to remove the lymph nodes. Unfortunately, 100% of the breast glands can never be removed. Even though mastectomy substantially reduces the chance of a later breast cancer, a small risk remains.

If a mastectomy is chosen, it may be psychologically advantageous to some women to do an immediate reconstruction (Chapter 34). 'Subcutaneous mastectomy' is a procedure in which the breast tissue is cut out through a small incision under each breast but the nipple and skin of the breast are not removed. Studies have shown that this procedure actually leaves behind nearly 15% of the breast tissue, so the risk of breast cancer is not eliminated. If the decision is taken to use a surgical approach to breast cancer prevention, eliminating as much of the breast tissue as possible is the goal, so total mastectomy with or without reconstruction is preferred.

The normal breast

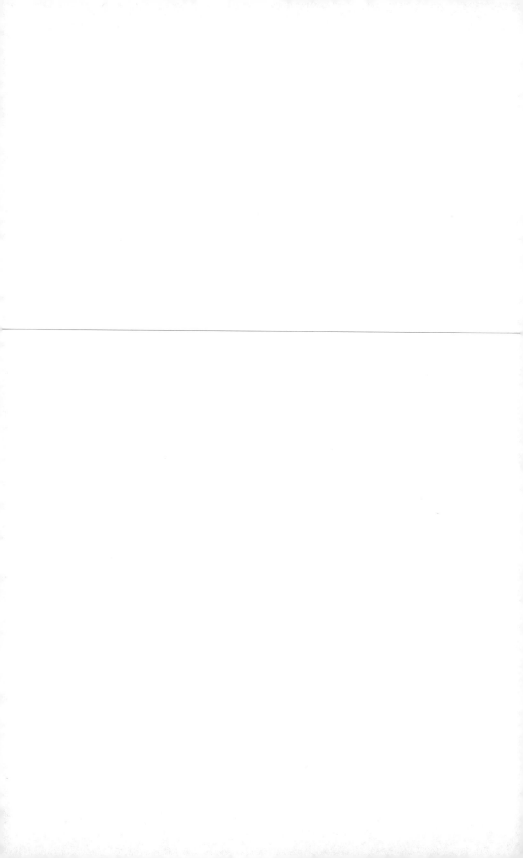

CHAPTER FIVE

Breast anatomy and function

MOST PEOPLE DON'T REALIZE how extensive the breast is. Breast tissue can be found as high as the collarbone (clavicle) and extends from almost the middle of the chest over the breastbone (sternum) to the armpit (axilla) (Figure 4).

What is in the breast?

The breast consists of milk glands, fat, fibrous tissue, blood vessels, nerves and tubes (ducts) that carry the milk to the nipple.

Breast milk is produced in hundreds of thousands of tiny glands (lobules) within the breast (Figure 5). These are drained by small ducts that collect the milk into larger glands which look like tiny bunches of grapes. From here, big ducts carry the milk to the nipple. The nipple surface contains about 20 duct openings, each draining a different part of the breast. All the milk glands are cushioned by fat. The normal 'lumps' that can be felt in your breast are a combination of the milk glands, fat and other fibrous tissues.

The proportion of milk glands, ducts and fat in the breast changes as a woman grows older. During puberty, and as the breast develops, it consists mainly of ducts. In a 20-year-old woman, most of the breast is made up of milk glands. During pregnancy and breastfeeding (lactation), the glandular content of the breast increases dramatically as the breast prepares to produce milk.

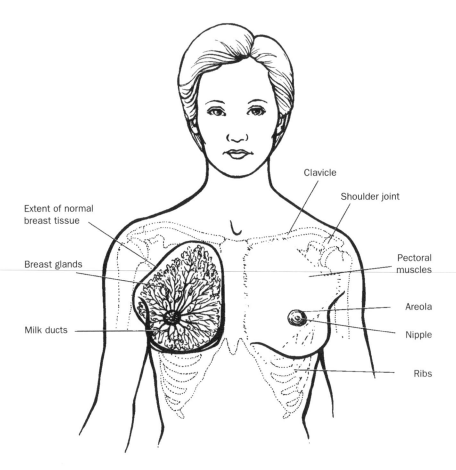

Clavicle

Shoulder joint

Extent of normal
breast tissue

Breast glands

Pectoral
muscles

Areola

Milk ducts

Nipple

Ribs

Figure 4: Extent of normal breast tissue and important underlying
structures.

The fat content increases as you age, especially after menopause.
In an elderly woman, almost all the breast is fatty tissue. Hormones
taken after menopause tend to maintain the glandular tissue and
delay the normal fatty replacement.

Ligaments help hold the breast in place

Throughout the breast there are many supporting ligaments,
like very thick, strong elastic bands, that connect onto the breast
bone or muscles under the breast. With age, these ligaments tend
to stretch and the normal breast begins to sag.

26

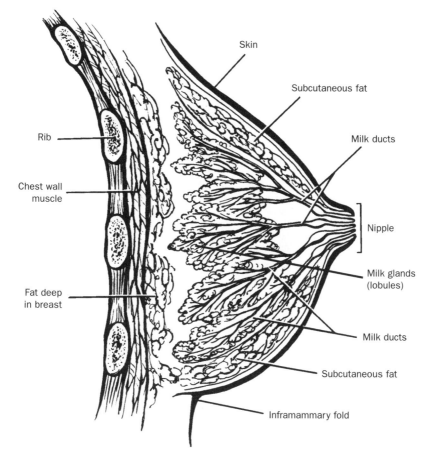

Skin

Subcutaneous fat

Milk ducts

Rib

Chest wall
muscle

Nipple

Milk glands
(lobules)

Fat deep
in breast

Milk ducts

Subcutaneous fat

Inframammary fold

Figure 5: A cross-sectional view of the breast showing the internal appearance of the breast and its relationship to the chest wall.

Muscles around the breast

A large, fan-shaped muscle lies beneath most of the breast. This is the pectoralis major muscle which is responsible for some of the shoulder and arm movements. If you tense your arm and 'push in' with your hand on your hip, you can feel this muscle as a firm ridge extending from the outside edge of the breast toward the armpit. The pectoralis minor muscle is smaller and not readily felt.

Lymph nodes: where infection fighting occurs

The purpose of the lymphatic system is to fight off infections in the body. There are tiny lymph vessels in every organ and tissue of the body. Fluid, which normally leaks from blood vessels to bathe body tissues, is collected by the lymph vessels and carried to groups of lymph nodes located in various places throughout the body. In the lymph nodes, infections are 'filtered out' and destroyed, and the 'treated' fluid then enters the blood stream.

Figure 6 shows the location of the main groups of lymph nodes that drain the breast. They are just above the armpit, above the

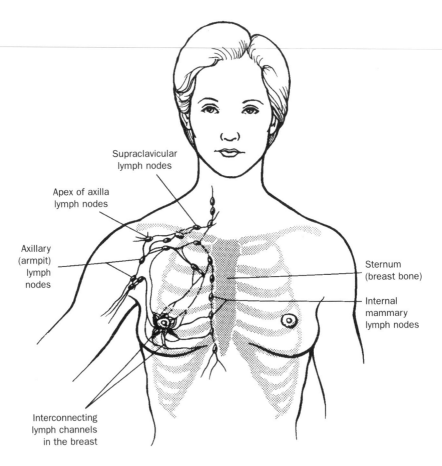

Figure 6: System of lymph nodes that drain the breast.

28

collarbone, and along the sternum (the internal mammary lymph nodes). There are about 30 lymph nodes in each armpit.

Lymph nodes are of particular importance in breast cancer because cancer cells sometimes enter the lymphatic vessels that drain the breast and can be carried to the lymph nodes where they settle and grow. In fact, the single most important factor in determining the future behavior of a breast cancer is if any cancer cells are found in the lymph nodes at the time of diagnosis (see Chapter 14).

Sensation and the nerves around the breast

Many nerves pass through the breast to the skin and to the nipple. In addition, the intercostal-brachial nerves come from the area between the ribs, through the armpit (axilla) and reach to the underside or back of the upper arm. These nerves are often stretched or cut during surgery in the armpit which leads to an unpleasant tingling, burning, numb or 'thick' sensation on the back or underside of the upper arm. These sensations usually fade partly or completely over several months after surgery, but some numbness is often permanent.

Routine methods for detecting breast cancer

CHAPTER SIX

Options for breast screening

SCREENING IS THE USE OF A TEST to detect disease early in an otherwise healthy individual. The goal of screening for breast cancer is to reduce the number of women dying from breast cancer by finding cancers that are so small they have not had a chance to spread beyond the breast. Such cancers are often too small to feel and may be cured by effective surgery.

Are screening mammograms useful?

A lot of research has examined different screening tests including mammograms and breast self examination (BSE), but there continues to be controversy about which screening test(s) should be used, how often and by whom. Increasing evidence suggests that if women age 50 to 79 years, (and possibly women ages 40 to 49 years) have a high-quality mammogram (x-ray of the breast) at least every two years it will reduce the woman's chance of dying from breast cancer by about one-third. This sounds like a large benefit but it needs to be put into context. Overall, for a healthy woman without a previous diagnosis of breast cancer, the lifetime chance of dying from breast cancer is about 4%. Therefore, on a population basis, regular screening will result in only a small improvement in the overall number of deaths each year. However, for the woman who has a small cancer detected by a screening mammogram, the benefit may be significant.

The chance of developing breast cancer, and therefore the value of screening mammograms, increase with age. A first mammogram will find approximately two cancers per 1000 women screened in their 40's, five cancers per 1000 women screened in their 50's and 10 cancers per 1000 women screened in their 70's. Screening mammograms can find small cancers (on average about 1.4 cm diameter), many of which are too small to feel. Such cancers have a much higher survival rate than cancers found when they are large enough to be felt by the woman or her doctor. As women age, other health problems play an increasing role in their lives. If a woman's life expectancy is less than 10 years, she is unlikely to benefit from the detection of a cancer before it can felt.

How often should women have screening mammograms?

Ongoing studies continue to examine how frequently healthy women should have routine screening mammograms. Current evidence suggests that about every two years is optimal. Doing mammograms more frequently substantially increases the cost of a screening program for little or no gain, while doing mammograms at intervals beyond three years may miss finding a developing cancer while it is still small and highly curable.

Other imaging tests, such as breast ultrasound or MRI scans, while useful in the diagnosis of women with specific breast problems, have not been proven worthwhile for screening otherwise healthy women in the general population. Such tests might be advisable for women with a very high risk of breast cancer (see Chapter 41, Hereditary cancer) or for women with very dense breasts where mammograms are much less helpful.

What about women less than age 50 years or over 79 years?

There is still controversy about screening women ages 40 to 49 years as the risk of breast cancer is lower and many such women have dense breasts. Mammograms are not as effective in detecting cancers in dense breasts compared to the more fatty breasts of older women. Some screening programs (for example, in British Columbia and the USA) invite women age 40 to 49 years to participate. Other programs require a doctor's referral at this age. Women younger than 40 years may benefit from screening if they are at very high risk on the basis of their family history. Mammogram screening before the age of 40 years should only be done after a careful discussion with an informed doctor. (See Chapter 41, Hereditary cancer.) Women older than 79 years are increasingly likely to have other health problems just because of their age. However, a healthy woman in her 80's who is likely to live another 10 years could benefit from continued breast screening.

Should women be taught Breast Self Examination?

Carefully conducted, large research studies have shown that women taught to perform breast self examination (BSE) did not have smaller cancers and had no better chance of survival if they were diagnosed with breast cancer, compared to women who were not taught BSE. As a result, regular BSE is falling out of favor as a screening test. However, many women find the breast cancer themselves and although BSE is not proven to reduce mortality, women who choose to do it should be informed how to do it effectively. Women who have had a cancer of one breast are at risk of a recurrence in that breast and for developing cancer in the second breast. The risk of developing cancer in the other breast is approximately 3% to 5% over 10 years. Women with a previous breast cancer therefore may be particularly motivated to do BSE. For assistance in learning how to do BSE, ask your nurse or doctor at the cancer center or contact the Cancer Information Service in your area. In addition, for an illustration of a suggested BSE technique see Appendix.

What are the limitations of screening?

Not all breast cancers can be found by a mammogram. Even more cancers are missed by BSE. Failure to detect cancer may occur because the cancer is the same density as the woman's normal breast glands or the cancer is so far to the edge of the breast that it is missed by the mammogram. Approximately 25% of breast cancers in women age 40 to 49, 15 % in women age 50 to 59 and 10% in women older than 60 will not be visible on a screening mammogram. For these women, even though a cancer is developing in the breast, the mammogram is 'negative.' A concern with these 'false negatives' is that they may lead to false reassurance. A woman could delay seeking medical help for a new lump if she has recently had a 'negative' mammogram.

Another downside of screening is that many women have 'false-positives'. This means that the mammogram is reported to be 'abnormal' when in fact no cancer is present. False positives occur in 10% to 15% of woman on a first mammogram and 5% to 7% of women having a second or subsequent mammogram. The lower rate on repeat mammograms is because the radiologist has the first one for comparison. Women with an abnormal test get alarmed and will have additional tests to determine if the abnormality is cancer of a 'false-positive'. These tests may be uncomfortable, costly and time consuming and many women live in fear of cancer while the additional tests are being done. Only approximately 5% of women with an abnormal screening mammogram will turn out to have a breast cancer.

Some cancers are discovered by routine physical examinations by doctors or nurses. Compared to mammograms or women finding cancers themselves, however, relatively few breast cancers each year are detected this way. An annual examination with your family physician should include examination of both breasts, the lymph node areas in the axilla (armpits) and above the collar bones. Any persistent or new lump or change in your breast should be investigated, even if a screening mammogram is 'negative' or normal.

What do I do when I find a lump?

CHAPTER SEVEN

A *visit to the doctor*

Finding a lump

THE DISCOVERY OF A NEW BREAST LUMP understandably causes tremendous anxiety. It may help to know that nearly 80% of lumps are benign (not cancerous). However, noticing a lump is often the first sign that may lead to a diagnosis of breast cancer. It is important to show any new lump or other breast abnormality to your doctor—and you should expect that it will be looked at in some detail.

What happens when I show the lump to a doctor?

The doctor will ask when you first noticed the lump and whether it has changed, especially in relation to your menstrual cycle. Any previous breast problems and risk factors will be discussed, including biopsies, infections or injuries, and facts regarding your menstrual cycle, use of medications or hormones, and your family history (health of family members).

It is best to examine the breasts of a premenopausal woman a week or two after the menstrual period, but if there is a worrisome lump you should not delay that first visit. During the breast examination you and the doctor are usually alone in the examining room, but you may request the presence of a nurse or bring a family member or friend along for moral support and as a 'second set of ears' to help remember what has been said.

You will be asked to disrobe at least the upper half of your body. Depending on your physician's judgement, you may have a partial or complete physical examination. This may include listening to your chest and examining the lymph node areas in your neck and armpits, both breasts and the abdomen. A pelvic examination is part of a yearly health exam and may be done but it is not essential to the diagnosis of breast cancer.

What happens next?

Depending on what the doctor thinks about the abnormality you may need no further tests. The doctor's recommendation will depend partly on your age. This is a factor that greatly affects the risk of getting breast cancer (Chapter 3). If you are in your teens, the breast lump is almost certainly benign: breast cancer is very rare in this age group. If you are in your twenties, the vast majority of lumps are benign, but an occasional case of breast cancer is seen every year. In the thirties and forties, breast cancer becomes more frequent, and among postmenopausal women there is a substantial possibility that a new breast lump is cancerous.

If some tests are needed, they may be done in the office or you may be sent for a mammogram, ultrasound or other tests. Assessment of your particular breast problem may require consultation with a surgeon, or you may need a biopsy, which involves removal of some tissue for further examination either with a small needle or by surgery (see Chapter 10). If the lump persists or grows, a biopsy may be considered even if the mammogram and ultrasound are normal.

CHAPTER EIGHT

Breast lumps and
other signs of trouble

Breast cysts

MANY WOMEN EXPERIENCE PAIN, lumpiness and swelling of the breasts. Such women are often described as having 'fibrocystic' disease. The tender, lumpy-feeling tissue may be completely normal, or may contain fluid-filled lumps called cysts that account for the lumps. As a woman's hormones change through the menstrual cycle, the fluid-filled cysts may become intermittently enlarged and tender especially in the days before a menstrual period begins.

As a rule, cysts do not turn into cancer. However if a biopsy is done and the cells lining the cysts or ducts show excessive cell growth (hyperplasia) and an abnormal appearance under the microscope (atypia), there is a higher risk of breast cancer developing (See Chapter 2). Any new change in the breast, especially if it involves only one side, may be a sign of cancer and should be checked carefully by a doctor. This change may be a lump or may be a thickening. Breast infections are rare except when breast feeding. Changes in the skin such as redness, or swelling of the breast in a woman who is not breast feeding, should be checked by a doctor.

Breast changes may indicate cancer

Breast lumps

There is no absolute way to describe how a cancerous lump is different from a non-cancerous or benign lump. Some women say that they knew it was different from other lumps they had felt in the past. Cancer lumps are usually firm or hard. They are generally painless but may be tender or sore. Not all cancers are lumps—some appear as 'thickenings' or 'ridges' but generally, thickened areas are caused by benign (not cancer) changes. Sometimes women first notice a lump in the armpit—an enlarged lymph node. Lumps that feel as though they are attached to the skin or also have skin redness are especially likely to be cancerous.

Nipple changes

Crusting, ulceration or eczema (weeping) of the nipple that does not go away in a few days may be the result of breast cancer cells growing into the nipple. This can be due to cancer or to another condition called Paget's disease in which cancer cells grow between the skin cells of the nipple (see Chapter 13). If the nipple becomes inverted (turns inward) it may be a sign of a growing cancer pulling on the ligaments of the breast as it enlarges.

Discharge from the nipple

A small amount of clear or whitish discharge can be squeezed from the nipple of most women and is NOT a cause for concern. If a discharge occurs on it own, spontaneously and is from a particular milk duct, it should be discussed with your doctor. If the discharge is bloody, it is usually due to a small, benign growth (a papilloma) in one of the milk ducts. However sometimes an early cancer may show up as bleeding from one nipple. A bleeding discharge should be investigated by your doctor and may require surgical removal of the bleeding milk duct.

Breast pain

Most often, no specific cause can be found for breast pain. However, a new, persistent localized area of pain or pain associated with a lump should not be ignored in the mistaken belief that breast cancer cannot be painful.

Changing breast size and skin changes

Occasionally one breast may become larger or swollen. The skin or nipple may show dimpling, redness or thickening. These changes are particularly worrisome because they could indicate that cancer has already spread and is blocking the drainage of the breast tissues to the lymph nodes.

CHAPTER NINE

Diagnostic mammograms, ultrasounds, MRI scans and PET scans

Diagnostic mammograms

A MAMMOGRAM IS AN X-RAY of the breast. When a new lump is found, a diagnostic mammogram should be taken of BOTH breasts. This allows evaluation of the lump and a routine check of the rest of that breast and also the opposite breast for unsuspected abnormalities. Each breast is flattened or compressed first from top-to-bottom and then from side-to-side, between the plastic plates of the mammogram machine as shown in Figure 7. Additional magnification and compression views may be taken to highlight parts of the breast that look suspicious or are not seen completely in the standard views. For example, an image may be taken to focus on the extreme outside part of the breast or if there appears to be a localized lump. Some apparent 'lumps' are due to overlapping of gland areas in the breast. With additional localized compression, the area is spread out and the 'lump' may disappear, proving that it is not cancer.

Signs of cancer on a mammogram

There is no single feature on a mammogram that always indicates cancer. However, there are features that are suggestive of cancer: a lump with jagged edges, clusters of irregular, tiny, white dots

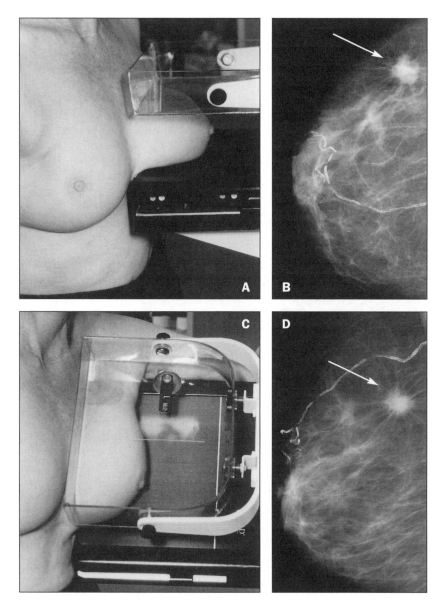

Figure 7: Localizing a breast abnormality requires two views, one from the top and one from the side of the breast. When the mammogram is taken with the breast flat (panel A) the x-rays pass from top to bottom through the breast to produce the image in panel B). Xrays passing from side-to-side though the breast (panel C) produce the image in panel D). The arrow identifies the cancer on the mammograms B and D.

that indicate calcium deposits, at pattern of tissue that looks like spokes on a wheel, and thickening of the overlying skin.

There are several possible reasons, other than cancer, for lumps or calcium deposits on a mammogram. If a lump or calcium deposit is very smooth and round or unchanged for several years, it is probably not cancer and doesn't need to be removed. However, if an abnormality is new or irregular, it should be biopsied to check if a cancer is present. Therefore, expert interpretation is necessary, and radiologists may seek a second opinion from a colleague before recommending a biopsy.

Other information from the mammogram

How big is the lump or cancer?

The mammogram can give information about the size of the lump or cancer. Calcifications, for instance, can sometimes be seen to extend many centimeters from the lump that you actually feel. If the lump turns out to be cancer, this information will be relevant in deciding whether it is feasible to save the breast. It is important, therefore, to have a mammogram to obtain this information before a biopsy is done because the breast may feel too bruised or sore to obtain a mammogram after the biopsy. Also, the bruise from a biopsy may cause confusion reading the mammogram: it can make a non-cancerous lump look suspicious.

Is there another 'hidden' cancer?

If one cancer is found, it is also important to check the rest of the breast and the breast on the opposite side to make sure that an additional hidden (occult) cancer is not missed. One or two women in 100 who are diagnosed with a breast cancer will be found to have a cancer in the other breast at the same time.

Are there different kinds of mammograms?

Diagnostic mammograms are done to closely examine an abnormality found during screening or as a new lump or change in the breast. Extra views may be taken of the area of concern including magnified views to more clearly define the area and decide if it looks sufficiently suspicious for cancer that a biopsy is needed. Screening mammograms (see Chapter 6) are generally two views of each breast and are done in healthy women with no apparent abnormality in their breasts with a goal of detecting small, early breast cancers before they can be felt. Digital mammography machines may be used for either diagnostic or screening mammograms. This technology is becoming more widely available. It enables the mammogram image to be more easily stored and analyzed and can even be sent remotely. One recent study has suggested that digital mammograms may be better able to find small cancers in young women with very dense breasts.

Mammograms do not show all cancers but if done properly and read by an experienced radiologist the majority of cancers are visible.

Ultrasound

A mammogram can show a lump but it cannot tell if the lump is a solid cancer, a solid benign tumor (such as a fibroadenoma) or a cyst (fluid filled cavity—usually benign). An ultrasound may be helpful in telling the radiologist if a lump is a cyst or a malignant appearing solid mass. Ultrasound uses sound waves rather than x-rays to assess the breast.

The ultrasound machine includes a small hand-held device that is pressed against the skin while sound waves are transmitted painlessly through the breast. Lubricating jelly is put on the skin to better transmit the sound waves through the skin surface. The sound waves are transmitted through the breast tissue and bounce back to the ultrasound machine. The machine then converts the pattern of rebounding sound waves into images which appear on a television monitor.

What does ultrasound show?

The main purpose of ultrasound is to find out if a lump in the breast is either solid (composed of tissue), or a cyst (filled with fluid). If a lump meets the strict criteria for a simple cyst, we can be confident that it is not cancer. Simple fluid-filled cysts can be easily drained with a thin needle (smaller than the needles used to take a blood test) if it is tender or large but usually a simple cyst can safely be left alone.

Not all cysts look completely typical on an ultrasound. If a cyst is partly solid, a 'core needle' or surgical biopsy may be done. An ultrasound may also show that a lump is solid or partly solid. Most

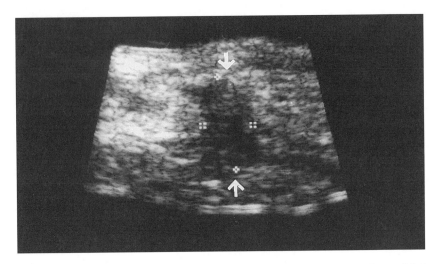

Figure 8: This ultrasound shows the characteristic 'taller-than-wide' orientation of a cancer (between the white arrows). Not all cancers are taller than they are wide, but virtually all masses with this appearance are cancer.

solid lumps are not cancer although this varies with the age of the woman. Several non-cancerous types of lumps occur frequently, the most common being fibroadenomas. If a fibroadenoma is confidently diagnosed by its appearance (and sometimes with a needle biopsy), surgical removal is not required.

Cancers are usually solid and have an irregular outline. The clue on the ultrasound that virtually always indicates that a lump is cancer is when the mass looks 'taller than wide' (Figure 8).

Ultrasound can also be used to direct a needle into a breast lump so that cells or small pieces of tissue can be removed to be examined under the microscope. This is called an ultrasound-guided needle biopsy. When ultrasound guidance is used to position the needle, the placement is more precise than when the needle is placed by finger guidance alone, especially if the lump is deep in the breast. When using ultrasound guidance, a negative or non-diagnostic result is virtually equivalent to a diagnosis of 'not cancer'. However, if there is a persistent, suspicious mass on the mammogram or ultrasound, it should be removed surgically, even if the needle test does not find any cancer cells.

Magnetic Resonance Imaging (MRI)

Magnetic Resonance Imaging (MRI) gives a different type of picture (image) than a regular x-ray or mammogram and there is no radiation involved. MRI scans have been used for other parts of the body for many years but breast MRI has only recently become more common. An MRI uses powerful magnets to create images before and after the intravenous injection of a material (gadolinium) that makes small cancerous (and some non-cancerous) tissue become more easily visible. MRI has a very high sensitivity, even in dense breasts where mammograms are sometimes not very helpful. However, areas that look abnormal on the MRI are frequently not cancer. Many normal areas may appear abnormal on the MRI. A highly skilled radiologist can often tell the difference between benign and cancerous changes but still, approximately 10% to 25% of women who do NOT have breast cancer will have something abnormal reported on a breast MRI scan. This can lead to concern that cancer may be present and may prompt additional tests including biopsies.

Studies have shown that MRI screening is helpful for women who carry an inherited mutation that predisposes them to develop breast cancer. Such women have a very high risk of developing breast cancer (See Chapter 43, Hereditary Cancer) and may benefit from regular breast screening with MRI in addition to mammograms. However, routine MRI screening of the general population, without inherited mutations, is not recommended.

MRI may also be helpful in diagnosis when the mammogram and ultrasound do not provide enough information, such as when the cancer first shows up in an axillary (armpit) lymph node with no disease found in the breast or after surgery when questions arise about whether all the cancer was removed. MRI is also useful in other situations such as monitoring the response to therapy of locally advanced cancer or in follow-up after lumpectomy plus radiation therapy when there are unusual changes in the breast scar.

Positron Emission Tomography (PET) scans

Positron emission tomography (PET) uses a small dose of radioactive-labeled glucose (sugar) to create an image of the extent of cancer in the body. This can sometimes be helpful in telling how far the cancer has spread. A small dose of radioactive glucose is injected into a vein and the scan is taken a short time later. Cells in the body that have a high metabolic activity (growing rapidly or consuming a lot of energy) concentrate the glucose and show up as a dark spot on the scan. Many invasive cancers are rapidly growing compared to their surrounding tissues and show up as 'hot' on the PET scan. If the cancer has spread to lymph nodes or other organs such as the lung, bone or liver, the PET scan may show 'hot spots' in these other organs. However, to be visible on a PET scan, the cancer lump generally has to be larger than half a centimeter ($1/4$ inch). Small microscopic clusters or individual cancer cells do not show up on a PET scan. Also, not all cancers, even when large, show up on a PET scan. Low grade, slow growing cancers are especially likely to have a 'negative' PET scan.

Research is being done with different types of injectible substances and specific types of breast cancer to understand how this powerful imaging technique can best be used in breast cancer. Machines that combine CT and PET are being used to more accurately localize actively dividing cancer within the body.

CHAPTER TEN

Biopsies

What is a biopsy and when is it needed?

IN MANY CASES, MAMMOGRAMS AND ULTRASOUND (see Chapter 9) give enough information to diagnose a benign condition in the breast and no further tests are necessary. However, if the diagnosis is still uncertain, then the next step is to take some breast tissue from the area and look at it under a microscope. The process of removing the cells or tissue is called 'taking a biopsy.' There are several ways to do this, some of which are quick and relatively painless, and others which are more complicated and require surgery.

A fine needle biopsy

A fine needle biopsy (or fine-needle aspiration biopsy) can be done in the doctor's office. It takes only a few seconds and usually causes no more pain than having a blood test. The skin may or may not be 'frozen' with a local anesthetic. Then, while holding the lump between two fingers, the surgeon or pathologist uses a syringe with a very thin needle to draw out some material from the lump (Figure 9). A fine-needle biopsy may also be done by a radiologist using ultrasound to ensure that the needle is accurately positioned in the lump.

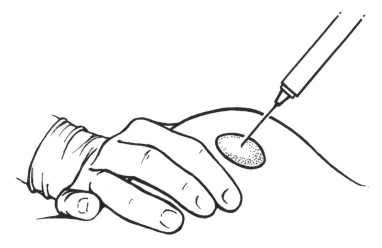

Figure 9: A needle biopsy involves the use of a needle to remove some material from the lump. The needle can be directed into the lump by feel or with ultrasound guidance (see Chapter 9).

If the lump is a cyst

If the lump is a cyst, the fluid in the cyst will be drawn into the syringe and the lump will disappear. No further action may be necessary! The cyst fluid may be a wide range of colors: clear, green, white, yellow, etc. Since little information can be obtained from this fluid, it is usually discarded. If the cyst fluid is bloody or if the lump remains even after all the fluid has been drained, there is cause for concern. In these cases, additional investigation is needed because there may be a cancer that is producing the cyst fluid or the lump. Also, if a cyst appears benign but keeps coming back after several aspirations (removal of fluid by needle), a surgical biopsy is advisable.

If the lump is solid

If the lump is solid, small clumps of cells (invisible to the naked eye) will be drawn into the needle. These cells are smeared onto slides or added to a jar with fluid and then prepared for the microscope. The preparation and interpretation of the slides may take from one to seven days.

Based on this microscopic examination of the cells a report will be issued that the aspiration was either 'positive', 'negative' or 'non-diagnostic'. If the report is 'positive for cancer' the diagnosis is correct 95% to 97% of the time. However, if the report is 'negative for cancer' or 'non-diagnostic,' it could just mean that the cancer was missed by the needle or that cancer cells, although present, were not removed during the aspiration. The fine needle biopsy results must be combined with the other tests performed about the mass including the physical examination, mammogram and ultrasound. If all these tests are benign, then it is rare that the abnormal area is cancer. But, if any one of the tests are suspicious, then further testing and even removal of the lump may be indicated.

A core biopsy

For a core biopsy, a needle is used to obtain multiple small cores of tissue about 2 mm in diameter and 1 to 3 cm in length. The needle is slightly wider than a fine-needle, but after local anesthetic (freezing) is given, the needle feels virtually the same as the smaller needle. The core biopsy needle works by using a spring to advance the needle into an abnormal area to cut small slivers of tissue, similar in size to flakes of coconut. After the local anesthetic is injected, a small 'nick' is made in the skin and the needle is inserted into the breast. When the samples are obtained, the spring makes a loud 'snapping' sound. Core biopsies are usually performed using ultrasound or mammographic guidance. To use mammographic guidance requires a special machine called a stereotactic unit attached to the mammogram machine and a special device to do the core-needle biopsy. Some stereotactic units are designed for the patient to lay on her tummy with her breast hanging through a hole in the table. Others have the patient seated or laying on her side. Core biopsies are being used more frequently as they reduce the number of unnecessary surgical biopsies and help in more accurate planning for the final surgery. Newer techniques using a vacuum attached to the core needle biopsy equipment allow larger areas of the breast to be removed without leaving a surgical scar.

A surgical (open) biopsy

A surgical biopsy or open biopsy involves making a small cut or incision in the skin of the breast and cutting out a piece of breast tissue (Figure 10). This usually takes place in a hospital, and can

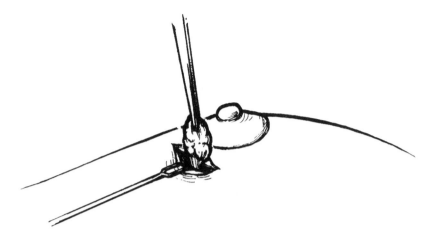

Figure 10: An open biopsy involves making a small cut in the skin and cutting out a piece of breast tissue.

be done under a local or general anesthetic. More and more open surgical biopsies have been replaced by core needle biopsies but in circumstances where a breast abnormality is not suitable for needle biopsy, an open biopsy may still be required.

Excisional biopsy: the whole lump is taken out

In addition to removing the entire lump, a small rim of the surrounding normal breast tissue is also removed. This leaves a small scar, but unless the lump was large relative to the size of the breast, it should not form a defect in the shape of the breast. Although such a biopsy can be a frightening experience, it is actually quite a simple surgical procedure.

Incisional biopsy: only a part of the lump is removed

Using anesthetic, the surgeon makes an incision through the skin and removes only a small part of the lump rather than the whole thing. This is done only when a lump is very large and when an excisional biopsy would cause a severe breast deformity or would not remove all of the cancer anyway. For example, when a cancer has invaded the skin or the chest wall, the doctor may do an incisional biopsy to confirm the diagnosis of cancer before discussing treatment options.

Other considerations

Generally, most suspicious masses should have a core needle biopsy as the first step to obtain tissue for diagnosis. However, if the lump needs to be removed for diagnosis using an open biopsy, it should be performed by a surgeon experienced in breast cancer surgery. The advantage is that the surgeon can assess the breast carefully and plan the position of the biopsy scar in such a way that it will fit with any additional surgery. The incision should always be placed to give the best cosmetic result and to make as little change in the shape of the breast as possible. The length of the biopsy scar will depend on the size of the lump, but it should not be more than a few centimeters long.

Whichever type of surgical biopsy is done, the specimen is sent directly to the pathologist for a number of studies (see Chapter 12).

A frozen section biopsy

In some situations a quick decision must be made about treatment while in the operating room, and a 'frozen section' or 'quick section' is done. This means that a piece of breast tissue is frozen while the patient is still on the operating table and ultra-thin slices of the tissue are examined under the microscope. This takes about 10 to 20 minutes. The problem with this method is that it is neither as good nor as complete as the diagnosis made when the pathologist has more time to examine the entire tissue sample and look at sections from several different areas of the tissue. The diagnosis of cancer inside the milk ducts can be especially difficult to make on a frozen section. Frozen sections are not performed as frequently today as they were in the past. The only reason to do a frozen section would be if the result found by the pathologist was going to have an immediate impact on the operation.

In cases where a diagnosis of cancer has not been made before the operation, it is usually best to perform the surgical biopsy and then wait for the pathologist to give a definite diagnosis, even if this takes a few days. Then, decisions about further tests and treatment can be made when the patient is awake and fully able to participate.

CHAPTER ELEVEN

If the screening mammogram is abnormal

What happens if my screening mammogram is abnormal?

IF YOU ARE TOLD THAT YOUR screening mammogram is abnormal do NOT assume that you have cancer! An abnormal result simply means that you need further evaluation to find out if the abnormality is really a cancer or some other problems such as scarring or cysts.

The first step is to see your doctor and to repeat the physical examination. Sometimes the abnormality can also be felt. A radiologist should compare the new mammogram to other mammograms you may have had previously. If it was the first time you had a mammogram in a new office, inform the technologist where you had your previous mammogram(s). Better yet would be to get the previous mammograms yourself and bring them to the new appointment.

A mass that has been present and unchanged for many years does not need to be removed. Often, more mammograms will be taken to provide greater detail of the abnormality (see Chapter 9). An ultrasound may be used to distinguish between a cyst or a solid mass. Also, a fine-needle or core biopsy done under ultrasound guidance or stereotactic control may provide more information (see Chapter 10).

Fine-wire localization biopsy

If the mass in your breast is still questionable after the physical examination, mammograms, ultrasound, and in most cases, fine-needle or core biopsies, it will have to be removed by surgical (open) biopsy so it can be examined in more detail. It would also have to be removed if the needle biopsy showed cancer. However, if the surgeon cannot feel the abnormal area, it becomes difficult to judge how much of the breast tissue to remove. A technique called 'fine-wire localization directed biopsy' can be used to help the surgeon find the exact location of the lump in the breast.

Before the surgery another mammogram or ultrasound is taken. With the breast still held between the mammographic plates or using the ultrasound for guidance, the radiologist locates the abnormality, and a thin, hollow needle is inserted into the breast and into the abnormal area. Subsequently, a very fine wire with a tiny hook on the end is threaded through the hollow needle and the needle is withdrawn, leaving the tiny hook at the end of the wire snagged near the suspicious area. The other end of the fine wire is sticking out of the skin (Figure 11). The patient is then taken to surgery for the open biopsy and the surgeon can follow the wire to find the area that needs to be removed. Depending on the type of abnormality that prompted the biopsy and the technique used to insert the fine-wire, an x-ray or ultrasound of the biopsy specimen may be done to confirm that the suspicious area has been removed (Figure 12).

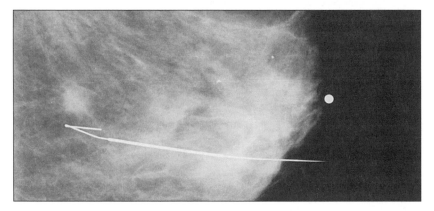

Figure 11: Guided by the mammogram, a fine wire with a hook on the end is placed through a needle into the vicinity of the suspicious area. At this stage the woman goes to the operating room for a biopsy.

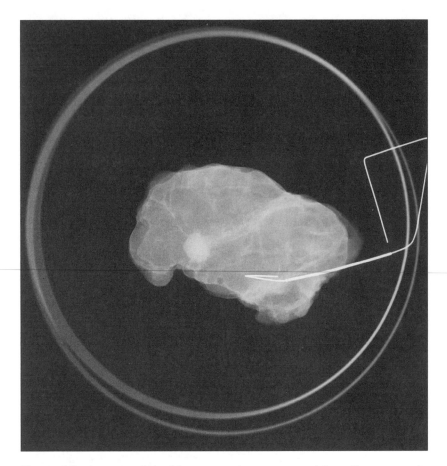

Figure 12: An x-ray of the biopsy specimen removed from the woman in Figure 11. The surgeon cut down along the wire until she reached the tip. She then removed the abnormal area and a margin of surrounding breast tissue. The abnormality turned out to be a 1 cm invasive ductal carcinoma with an excellent chance for cure.

SECTION FIVE

What type of cancer is it?

CHAPTER TWELVE

The pathology report:
Reading the cancer's telltale signs

WHEN A SURGEON REMOVES a suspicious lump from the breast, a lot of important information can be gained by looking at the lump itself and examining small bits of it under the microscope (Figures 13 and 14). This detailed examination establishes whether cancer is present or not. In situations where the diagnosis of cancer has already been made, it provides information that helps predict how the cancer will behave in the future. Is it likely to grow back? Where? When? With this information, a treatment strategy can be planned with the goal of preventing recurrence and maximizing your chance of being cured. Uncovering the information and reporting it is the role of the pathologist who is a physician specializing in the study of tissues. The pathologist's written summary is called the pathology report.

The three sections of the pathology report

The pathology report contains three main sections: the gross description of the tissues (as seen with the naked eye), the microscopic description and the summary (final diagnosis).

The gross description of the tissues

The pathologist reports on what he or she can see with the naked eye: the size of the lump, and the number and size of any

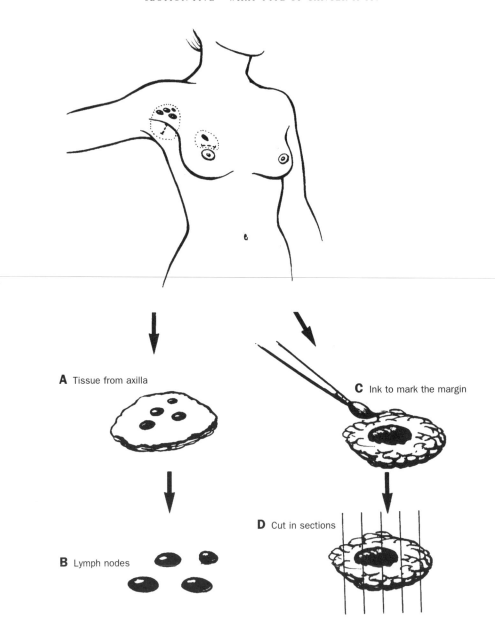

Figure 13: Tissue from the axillary dissection (A) is examined and any lymph nodes are removed and counted (B). The external surface of the breast tissue containing the cancer is painted with ink (C) and then the specimen is cut into sections (D).

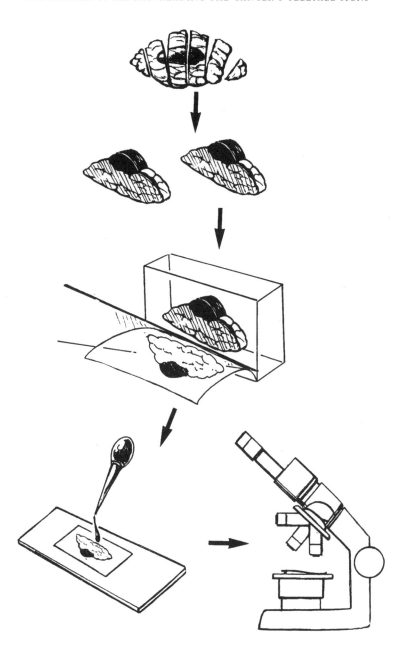

Figure 14: Preparation of a small piece of the breast lump for viewing on a microscope slide.

lymph nodes. It is then noted how close the cancer is to the edge of the specimen. This is important: if the cancer is right against the edge rather than being centered within a block of normal-looking tissue, there is a higher likelihood that some cancer cells may have been left behind in the breast. Once samples are cut for microscopic examination, the rest of the excised tissue is immersed in a container of formaldehyde and labeled with your name. Specimens are stored like this for years in case further examination is required.

The microscopic description

Under the microscope, breast cancer cells look different from normal cells. The pathologist will describe details of the type of cancer, the grade (an assessment of how aggressive the cancer looks), and whether the cancer has invaded the tissues surrounding the main cancer, especially whether cancer cells are seen within the lymph or blood vessels in the breast. The report should also include the amount of estrogen and/or progesterone receptor content in the cancer cells. As well the amount of activity (expression) of the HER2 gene (Human Epidermal Receptor 2; also written as her2-neu or c-erb-B2) is reported as negative or a level 1, 2, or 3 positivity for HER2. This may be important in patients to predict the cancer's behavior and to determine if the drug Herceptin® will be useful (see Chapter 28).

Another important feature is the number of mitoses—cells that have been 'caught in the act' of multiplying, which is an indicator of the cancer's growth rate.

If any lymph nodes have been removed from under the arm the pathologist will report on whether the cancer has spread into the lymph nodes. In fact, the report should document how many nodes were found, and how many, if any, were affected by cancer ('involved' or 'positive nodes'). It should also mention whether the cancer has grown through the lymph node and out into the surrounding fat (called extranodal or extracapsular extension).

Final diagnosis

This is a summary of the results of the gross and microscopic examinations. The process of tissue inspection and preparation of the report usually takes from two to seven days. The report then becomes a permanent part of the patient's record. The important features which usually influence your doctor's decision about treatment strategy are listed in Table 4.

Table 4	**Features of the pathology report that affect treatment strategy**

The Tumor

Size: measured in centimeters

Type: in situ, invasive, or mixed (see Chapters 13 and 14); ductal, lobular, or other

Invasion: of the lymphatic or vascular spaces

Grade: the degree of aggressiveness, includes assessment of the number of mitoses (dividing cells), the appearance of the cell nuclei and whether the cells are trying to form milk ducts

Necrosis (dying cells): a measure of the cancer's growth rate)

Receptors: for estrogen and/or progesterone

HER 2 status: negative or positive for gene overexpression

Extension of tumor: to skin, to muscle, to excision margins

Other prognostic markers: p53, ploidy, p27, oncogenes, other growth factors (these are not standard)

The Lymph Nodes

Total number of lymph nodes recovered

Number of involved nodes

Maximum size of involved nodes

Extranodal extension (growth beyond the lymph nodes): present or absent

CHAPTER THIRTEEN

In situ cancer: Cancer that hasn't invaded or spread

'IN SITU' CANCER IN THE BREAST refers to a cancer that is still within the milk ducts and/or lobules (the milk glands) of the breast. In other words, the cancer cells have not invaded through the walls of the milk ducts; they are in the same place (or situation) where they first formed.

Ductal carcinoma in situ (DCIS)

The milk ducts become blocked and enlarged as cancer cells accumulate inside them (Figure 15). Calcium tends to collect in the blocked ducts (Figure 16) and is visible on mammograms as tiny white lines and dots (Figure 17). These clusters of fine, irregular calcifications on a mammogram often indicate in situ cancer and, if present, a biopsy should be done. In situ cancer of the ducts accounts for 20% to 30% of the cancers found on screening mammograms. This type of cancer is also referred to as 'intraductal cancer.' Ductal carcinoma in situ, if left untreated, may progress to form an invasive cancer with the potential for spreading throughout the body (Figure 16). This progression can take as long as five to 10 years.

Ductal carcinoma in situ occurs as two different cell types, with one tending to progress to invasion more quickly than the other. The first type, which progresses more slowly, consists of smaller,

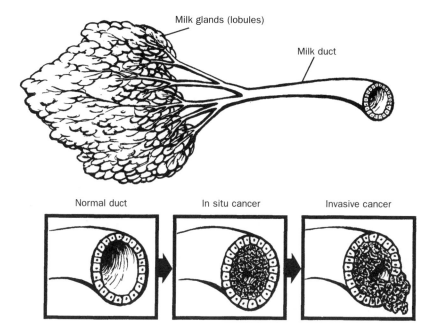

Figure 15: Cross-sectional view of milk duct. The duct may become filled with in situ cancer cells that eventually form an invasive cancer.

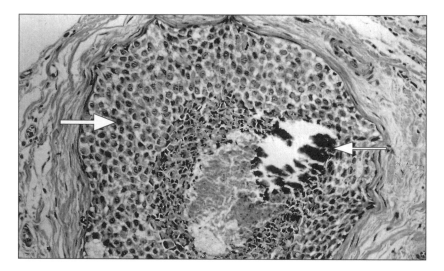

Figure 16: Ductal carcinoma in situ cells (large arrow) seen under the microscope. The dark material (small arrow) is a calcium deposit which has formed in an area of dead and dying cancer cells (necrosis).

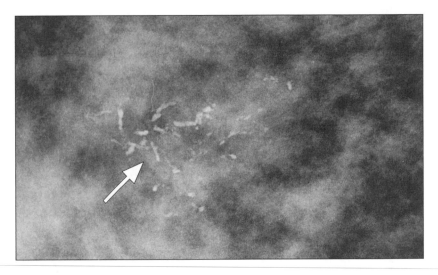

Figure 17: Calcium deposits typical of ductal carcinoma in situ as seen on a mammogram.

more normal-looking cells. These may be called 'solid,' 'papillary' or 'cribiform'. The second type, called 'comedocarcinoma,' often progresses to invasion early in its growth and consists of large, irregular-shaped cells. Because they are growing quickly, these cells tend to outgrow their supply of sugar and oxygen. As a result, cells in the middle of the ducts start to die (called necrosis) and eventually the body deposits calcium in the dead cells (Figure 17). It is crucial that comedocarcinomas are treated effectively. Ductal carcinoma in situ may be estrogen receptor positive or negative. Recent studies suggest that patients with estrogen receptor positive DCIS may benefit from the antiestrogen tamoxifen. Chapter 23 describes the treatment of in situ cancers.

Lobular carcinoma in situ (LCIS)

Lobular carcinoma in situ refers to cancer cells that have formed in the milk glands (rather than the milk ducts) and are still confined there. This type of in situ cancer is often found in women around the age of menopause. Lobular carcinoma in situ is different from ductal carcinoma in situ in that there is a high risk that the entire tissue of both breasts may develop cancer. Therefore, treatment of lobular carcinoma in situ (Chapter 23) must be aimed at both breasts rather than just the affected one, (unlike the case with ductal carcinoma in situ). Lobular carcinoma in situ is almost always hormonally responsive.

Paget's disease

Paget's disease is a rare form of in situ cancer that can occur in a 'pure' form but it is often accompanied by an invasive cancer. It is recognized when cancer cells invade the skin and make visible skin changes. Paget's disease appears as a reddish, itching, scaling or 'eczema' of the nipple caused by cancer cells in the skin of the nipple and areola. Although the traditional treatment is mastectomy, it may be possible to save the breast if there is no underlying invasive cancer. However, the breast must be large enough to tolerate the removal of skin, and the woman needs to accept that there will be a change in sensation and appearance due to the removal of the nipple and areola.

As well as removing the nipple and some surrounding skin, a sample of the breast tissue beneath should also be taken to make sure there is no accompanying invasive cancer. It is not yet clear whether radiation therapy should always follow surgical excision of Paget's disease, but in most cases, radiation treatment is added when using a breast-conserving approach to reduce the chance of cancer regrowth in the breast.

CHAPTER FOURTEEN

The different types of invasive cancer

What is invasive cancer?

CANCER CELLS HAVE TWO CHARACTERISTICS that are important. One is that cancer becomes invasive and cells can grow through the walls of the milk ducts and glands into the normal fatty tissue of the breast (Figure 15). The cells can continue to grow causing a lump or thickening.

The second characteristic is that the invasive cancer cells can also travel. These cells can be carried elsewhere in the body through the blood stream or lymphatic system. It is this ability to invade and spread through the body that makes us fear cancer. When cancer spreads to other parts of the body, we say it has 'metastasized' and the tumors growing in these areas away from the breast are called 'metastases'. If we look at these 'metastases' under the microscope, we would see that wherever they are in the body, they are actually breast cancer cells with the features of a breast cancer that was initially discovered in the breast.

Invasive cancers do not usually grow like an expanding balloon. Rather, finger-like projections of cells grow out into the normal breast tissue from the main cancer. These finger-like projections may be seen under a microscope and sometimes even on a mammogram. Figure 7 shows the typical appearance of an invasive cancer on a mammogram.

To try to determine how a cancer will behave in the future, the tumor is carefully assessed by the pathologist. Currently, cancers are divided into types according to their appearance under the microscope (the tumor histology). Using this classification, the classically recognized types of breast cancer are:

From Ducts and glands
Infiltrating Ductal Carcinoma
–Type not otherwise specified (75%)
   – tubular (1%)
   – mucinous (1%)
   – colloid (1%)
   – medullary (1%)
   – inflammatory (3-5%)
Lobular carcinoma (15%)
Squamous carcinomas (less than 1%)
Mixed carcinomas (adenosquamous and metaplastic cancers) (less than 1%)

From other parts of the breast
Cystosarcoma phylloides (1%)
Sarcomas (less than 1%)
Lymphomas (less than 1%)

Ductal carcinoma is the most common and is also called mammary carcinoma or infiltrating ductal adenocarcinoma. Lobular carcinomas, which account for about 15% of breast cancers, are usually estrogen dependent, often difficult to diagnose on a mammogram and have a slightly higher risk of being in both breasts.

Newer Classification Schemes

Recently it has become clear that a classification according to how cells look under the microscope, does not give enough information about how the cancer will behave in the future. Cells have genes and molecular markers that act as the 'engines' for the cell and determine how rapidly the cells will grow, whether they will spread and in some cases how they will respond to treatment. 'Molecular' classifications of tumors provide more information and may allow the oncologist to make more individualized treatment recommendations. Using both molecular and pathological features provides a better ability to predict a cancer's future behavior.

The current important molecular, pathological and clinical features to consider are:
1. Hormone Receptors: positive or negative
2. HER2 overexpression: present or absent

3. Tumor grade: Grade 1, 2, 3 (or low, moderate or high)
4. Extent of disease: limited or more extensive (see Chapter 16, Staging)
5. Other features

Hormone Receptors

Breast cancers are tested to see if they are sensitive to hormones. Approximately 75% of breast cancers have hormone receptors. Cancers that have hormone receptors respond to the female hormones, estrogen and progesterone. When stimulated with these hormones the tumor cells grow and divide. Estrogen receptors are the most common receptors and predict whether the tumor will respond to anti-estrogen therapy (see Chapter 30). Progesterone receptors are less common and seem to work with the estrogen receptor to make the cell more responsive to hormonal treatment.

HER2 overexpression

HER2 is a cancer gene. In 20-25% of breast cancers this gene is overexpressed, which means that there is too much HER2 in the cell. Studies have shown that breast cancers with HER2 overexpression behave in a more aggressive manner, growing more quickly and often traveling to other sites of the body. As well, studies have suggested that HER2 cancers may respond differently to some of our standard cancer treatments. A drug that specifically targets HER2 (trastuzumab or Herceptin®, see Chapter 39) is used for women with recurrent disease and has recently been shown to further reduce recurrence and improve survival when used in early breast cancer if the tumor was overexpressing HER2 (see Chapter 28).

Grade

When the pathologist examines the cancer under a microscope, a number of features are assessed which together help us predict how quickly the cancer will grow. Considering these features, the pathologist may use a grading system which gives the cancer a score. Some pathologists report grade on a scale of one to three and others on a scale of three to nine. Cancers may be low grade (score 1 out of 3, or 3-5 out of 9), moderate grade (score 2 out of 3, or 6-7 out of 9) or high grade (score 3 out of 3, or 8-9 out of 9). 'Low grade' refers to a slower growing cancer. 'Moderate' describes a medium growing cancer while a cancer that grows quickly is classified as 'high grade'.

Extent of disease at diagnosis: Limited versus more extensive

A number of features are used to determine this:

- Size: The larger the cancer, the more likely it is to spread. Breast cancers are classified as 'small' when they are up to two cm in diameter, 'medium' if they are between two and five cm and 'large' if they are bigger than five cm. If the cancer is invading into the skin or growing into the muscle or chest wall it is called 'locally advanced' and has a higher risk of recurring or spreading.
- Nodes: Cancer cells can travel and the first place they may spread is into the lymph nodes. The risk of the cancer spreading increases according to the number of armpit (axillary) lymph nodes that are found to have cancer. As well as the number of nodes involved, the risk may be related to the amount of cancer in the lymph node. The risk is higher if there are large lymph nodes filled with cancer compared to a tiny millimeter of cancer in one node. The cancer may also extend out from the lymph node into the fat in the armpit which may increase the risk of the cancer recurring in the armpit.
- Lymphatic or Vascular invasion: If cancer cells are found in the lymph channels or blood vessels in the breast, the prognosis is similar to the situation of having one to three cancerous lymph nodes.

Other Features

To more effectively predict how a cancer is going to behave, many researchers assess other features which can contribute extra information. These include a number of ways of assessing how quickly the cell is growing such as 'mitotic index', 'percent of S-phase' and 'ploidy'. Other molecular features such as the presence of genes p53, p27 and others are determined. In addition, some laboratories and companies are starting to look at a technique called 'microarray' which assesses a large number of genes that the breast cancer cell may 'over' or 'under' express. This means that a cancer may have too much or too little of a gene and this may affect how it grows. These tests may prove to be very important in the next few years but at this time are still not ready for everyday use.

Rare Types of Invasive Cancer

Inflammatory cancer

Inflammatory cancer is an aggressive form of cancer that presents with a red breast that looks like an infection. The cancer cells spread rapidly to the lymph channels in the breast and skin causing the breast to become swollen, enlarged, and tender and the skin to get warm and red. Any woman who appears to have a breast infection (other than women who are breast feeding and may get mastitis) should be checked promptly to exclude the possibility of inflammatory cancer. A mammogram may show thickening but the diagnosis is usually made with a biopsy.

Sarcomas

Sarcomas are tumors that come from connective tissue such as nerves, fat, fibrous tissue, or blood vessels of the breast rather than the milk ducts. Cystosarcoma phylloides may be benign or malignant depending on the number of cells that are seen dividing when the tumor is examined under the microscope. This tumor is usually cured by surgery with either a partial or full mastectomy depending on the size of the tumor and its location. It is important that it is completely removed as these tumors can cause problems by re-growing in the original site or on the chest wall.

PART TWO | **What are my options now that I have a diagnosis of breast cancer?**

An overview of treatment

CHAPTER FIFTEEN

An overview of breast cancer treatment

Is there more than one way to treat breast cancer?

YOU MAY FEEL CONFUSED to learn that the treatment recommended to you for breast cancer is different from what others have received. For example, your aunt may have had a mastectomy, while a friend was treated with chemotherapy and radiation first, followed by mastectomy while another friend might have had a 'lumpectomy,' radiation and tamoxifen.

Why all these different approaches? What do these different treatments mean? What is the best treatment for you?

When a breast cancer is diagnosed there are three major decisions to be made:

1. What to do regarding your breast: save it or remove it (mastectomy)
2. What to do regarding the lymph nodes in your armpit (nothing, surgery, radiation, or both surgery and radiation)
3. What to do regarding treatment of the rest of the body (nothing, chemotherapy, hormone therapy, Herceptin® or a combination of chemotherapy, Herceptin® and hormone therapy).

The answer to these issues will depend on the type and extent (or stage) of cancer (determined by tests), your ability to tolerate the treatments, and your preferences.

If the cancer is confined to the breast and lymph nodes in the armpit, the 'primary therapy,' is usually surgery (Chapter 19), aimed at removing the cancerous tissues. New treatments such as preoperative chemotherapy, also called 'neoadjuvant,' are being explored (Chapter 27), especially in cases where the tumor is bulky. The important decision about the type of surgery to be used, either mastectomy or an approach that saves the breast, requires your input (Chapter 20).

Once the cancer has been removed, the prognosis of the cancer can be determined from the pathologist's examination of the cancerous tissue (Chapters 12 to 14). A recommendation for additional treatment, called 'adjuvant therapy' (Chapter 22) is based on weighing the likelihood that your cancer will grow back after the surgery against the unnecessary side effects caused by too much treatment.

If the risk of regrowth in the 'local area' (breast or chest wall and lymph nodes) is substantial, then adjuvant radiation therapy is used (Chapter 25). To reduce the chance of recurrence elsewhere in the body, additional treatment with drugs (hormones, chemotherapy or Herceptin®; Chapters 28 and 30) is offered except to those women with the very lowest risk of recurrence. If recurrence in the local area and throughout the rest of the body are both a concern, combined types of adjuvant therapy may be recommended, for example, radiation together with chemotherapy and/or Herceptin® and/or hormonal therapy.

CHAPTER SIXTEEN

Staging and prognosis

What is staging?

AFTER THE DIAGNOSIS OF CANCER has been made it is important to determine the extent or 'stage' of the cancer before deciding on the treatment plan. Briefly, a cancer that is small and confined to the breast is at an early stage, and one that has spread to other parts of the body is advanced or metastatic. Based on knowledge of the extent of the disease, your surgeon or oncologist (cancer specialist) can make recommendations about the chances of being cured by surgery alone, the type of surgery that is likely to give you the best possible outcome, and whether additional treatments (radiation, hormones, chemotherapy or Herceptin®) will be helpful.

The physical examination

One of the most important investigations is the physical examination done by the surgeon or oncologist. Your lungs, liver, abdomen, back and limbs will be examined for abnormalities. Your breast will be examined and any lumps will be measured. Your armpit and neck will be felt to see if any lymph nodes are enlarged. Not all enlarged lymph nodes are cancerous: the doctor will try to determine this by assessing whether a node feels normal or enlarged, soft or hard, and whether it is movable. If a suspicious lymph node is found, a fine-needle aspiration may be done (see

Chapter 10). Unfortunately, simple physical examination of the armpit is not foolproof, and sometimes cancerous lymph nodes are not found until surgery.

Blood tests

Blood tests will be done to check whether your bone marrow, liver and kidneys are working normally. Some doctors also order blood tests to look for 'tumor markers,' which are proteins that leak out of cancer cells and can be measured in the blood. These markers are not reliable for diagnosing cancer, but occasionally suggest metastases. The markers that can be measured in breast cancer are CEA (carcinoembryonic antigen), CA15.3 (cancer antigen 15.3) and CA125.

Other tests

A chest x-ray should be taken to check the condition of the lungs and to check for any benign or malignant lung disease. For older women, an electrocardiogram (ECG) may be done to check the heart.

A bone scan is only necessary for women who have a high risk of metastasis to the bones, actual symptoms of such metastases or are being considered for a research study. The same goes for ultrasound examinations of the liver. A liver ultrasound is not done routinely.

Official systems of staging

There are several systems for classifying the extent or stage of breast cancer. The two most common are the Stage I, II, III, IV system (Table 5) and the TNM system (Table 6).

It is important to recognize that staging systems provide only rough estimates of the chances for survival. The numbers are just averages. They do not determine specific outcome or prognosis of any one particular woman. Each case is unique and other details of your own case, not just the size and location of tumor, are used to help determine your chance of being cured by surgery alone or with additional therapy. In other words, these staging systems, although important, are most useful for providing an approximate idea of the extent of disease to help plan the treatment strategy, but they are far too basic to determine an individual woman's outcome precisely.

82

Table 5 **Stage definitions (I to IV) of breast cancer**

Definition	Average five-year survival
Stage I Tumor 2 cm or less, no metastases, no cancer in lymph nodes	80% to 95%
Stage II Tumor 2-5 cm but not involving skin and chest wall. If lymph nodes are involved they must be movable	50% to 70%
Stage III Advanced local tumor, fixed to the skin or chest wall, or presence of lymph nodes 'attached' to structures in the axilla or enlarged above the collarbone	30% to 60%
Stage IV Cancer spread beyond the breast and axilla, to distant organs	5% to 20%

The Stage I, II, III, IV system

This simple system defines four stages of breast cancer (see Table 5). Stage I represents early cancer, with a small tumor and no spread to the lymph nodes in the armpit. In stages II and III, the tumor is progressively more advanced, while stage IV refers to metastatic disease that has spread to other areas of the body.

Since each stage (I to IV) is rather broad, the survival expectation within each stage is quite variable. For example, for a woman with stage I cancer, the average survival at five years after diagnosis is 85%. However, within this category there could be a woman with a mammographically-detected cancer of just 0.5 cm in diameter as well as another woman with a 2 cm diameter tumor and cancer invading the lymphatic vessels in the breast. The first woman would have a 95% chance of living free of cancer for over 10 years while the second woman would have a survival expectation closer to that of women with stage II tumors (a 30% to 50% chance of recurrence within five years with surgery alone).

Also, it must be noted that the 'grade' of the tumor refers to the appearance of the cancer cells under the microscope, not be confused with the 'stage' of the disease.

Table 6 **The TNM staging system**

TUMOR Stages: (T)

T(0):	no identifiable tumor in the breast
Tis:	in situ (noninvasive) cancer only
T(1a):	invasive cancer 5 mm or less in diameter
T(1b):	invasive cancer 6 to 10 mm in diameter
T(1c):	invasive cancer 11 to 20 mm in diameter
T(2):	invasive cancer 2 cm to 5 cm in diameter
T(3):	invasive cancer larger than 5 cm without skin or chest wall involvement
T(4a):	tumor of any size fixed to the chest wall
T(4b):	tumor of any size invading the skin
T(4c):	tumor of any size invading both chest wall and the skin
T(4d):	inflammatory cancer

NODE Stages: (N)

N(0):	no evidence of palpable lymph nodes
N(1):	palpable, mobile lymph nodes in the armpit only
N(2):	lymph nodes in the axilla are fixed to each other or to adjacent structures such as nerves, muscles, skin or bones
N(3):	involved lymph nodes beside the breast bone or above the collarbone

METASTASIS Stages: (M)

M(0):	no evidence of metastases
M(1):	metastases are present

The TNM system

The TNM system defines the extent of the cancer based on three features of the tumor: the size/extent of the tumor (T), lymph node involvement (N), and the presence or absence of metastases (M). There are nine possible 'T' categories, four 'N' categories, and two 'M' categories. This system is not as simple as the Stage I, II, III, IV system for everyday use, but it is useful for cancer specialists to communicate with each other.

CHAPTER SEVENTEEN

Strategies for navigating the cancer care system

THE TREATMENT OF BREAST CANCER involves many different health care providers. Most patients assume these people work as part of a well-coordinated team but, unfortunately, this is not often the case. Each professional is qualified in her or his field, but they often work in relative isolation.

Find a helper if you can

In most situations, there is no single person who functions in the role of 'case manager' to coordinate a patient's medical files and their passage through the treatment system. Many patients assume that their general practitioner (GP) will take on this role, but it is not a responsibility that many GPs can assume. Not all medical reports are automatically forwarded to the GP and, of those that are, some may be slow in arriving. In addition, even though breast cancer is the most common form of cancer in women, each GP will have only one or two patients with a new diagnosis of breast cancer each year. The GP may not feel well equipped to handle the details of the multiple options facing a woman with breast cancer. As a result, many patients find that they need someone, other than themselves, to act as a 'navigator' or 'case manager' to help them sift, organize, integrate and keep track of all the information, advice and appointments they encounter.

Some suggest that the patient herself would make the best case manager since she knows the most about her history and any special health problems. However, most cancer treatments subject the patient to a high degree of physical and psychological strain. Thus, the addition of case-management responsibilities to this load creates a huge additional burden. If possible, it is best to have a second person involved.

Typically, the person who takes on this role is a spouse, partner, relative or close friend. No medical background is necessary, although it helps. The most important thing is a willingness to devote the time and attention needed to help the patient.

To be most helpful, the case manager needs to accompany the patient to most, if not all, appointments, tests and procedures. Almost all health care providers will allow the case manager to stay with the patient if the patient asks. Page 87 lists some important pointers about the role of a case manager.

Questions to ask about drug or other therapy

When the patient has been prescribed a new drug or treatment as part of her breast cancer care, the case manager should ask specific questions of the physician, pharmacist, or nurse before the patient begins taking the drug. (These questions should also be asked of an alternative health care practitioner, such as a naturopath, who has prescribed alternative therapies, e.g. herbal remedies or vitamins.)

1. Why is this drug or treatment being prescribed?
2. What is the goal of the therapy? Is it for cure? Is it to slow disease? Is it to relieve symptoms?
3. Is this a standard or a new therapy? What is the evidence for using this particular protocol?
4. How and when do we know if the treatment is working? How long should it be continued?
5. What happens if the treatment doesn't work? Should it be stopped or the dose increased?
6. Are there other treatment options?
7. What are the potential harmful effects? How should we recognize and manage them?
8. Who should we call if there are problems or if we have more questions?

STRATEGIES FOR NAVIGATING THE CANCER CARE SYSTEM

A word about the Internet

Many patients and their case managers will have access to the Internet. The Internet is a mixed blessing because it contains almost as much potentially harmful information as it does helpful information. Your specialist or the librarian at your local cancer treatment center may be able to direct you to websites that provide credible information.

Helpful hints for the case manager

Some duties that a case manager could undertake with the patient's consent:

1. Take a note book and tape recorder to all appointments. (Ask the physician before turning on the tape recorder.)
2. Keep a written record of all the instructions to the patient.
3. Keep a record of all the tests that are ordered and appointments. This may avoid duplication of testing.
4. Ask for copies of all the medical and pathology reports. This is the patient's right under the freedom of information laws in most places. Keep them all in a binder. Understand these are used to record results and may not include instructions.
5. Speak up when you are becoming frustrated with information overload or conflicting information. If necessary, put your concerns in writing (tactfully and positively).
6. Carry a cell phone or pager if you can't be easily reached.
7. Remember that the patient's medical files are not routinely passed from one health care facility to another unless the patient or physician requests specific information. Ensure that the patient informs the health care provider of any special problems or conditions that have arisen since the last visit including new medications, allergy alerts or reactions to tests or anesthetics.
8. If possible, secure other sources of information and support from health care providers who are not directly involved with the patient's care. These people can be a valuable source of medical knowledge and insight.
9. Encourage the patient to have a good relationship with her family physician. Although the specialist will direct most of the cancer specific treatments, it is the family physician who

maintains contact with the patient when her cancer treatments are completed. As well, the family physician should receive results of tests and can be called to get results prior to the next appointment with the oncologist.

10. Before the patient sees a specialist such as a surgeon or oncologist, fax any questions you have. Because of their busy schedules, they may find it helpful to receive the questions in writing and in advance of the appointment.

11. The patient may want to invest in "call display" so she can answer only the calls that she chooses, while leaving the others for you to respond to when time allows.

12. Your responsibility is not to become a medical expert but an expert on what has happened (treatments, patient moods, test results, etc.) in relation to the patient.

13. Maintain a calm, caring presence for the sake of the patient and yourself.

14. Almost every health care provider is a skilled expert, but is probably overworked with more than the optimal number of patients. They are doing their best and your goal is to help them achieve this. Positive comments expressing your appreciation are most helpful.

15. Allow friends and relatives to help you and give you support. It is essential that you do not 'burn out' so consider your own needs and take good care of yourself.

The surgical options

Chapter Eighteen

The doctor has suggested surgery: What should I do?

TODAY'S OPERATIONS ARE MUCH LESS EXTENSIVE than in the past. When it comes to surgery, 'more' is not necessarily 'better'. Today, there is usually a team of experts who treat the cancer with a combination of surgery, radiation, chemotherapy, hormones and Herceptin®. You are also part of the team and have a role to play—learning about the disease, hearing the options, discussing your needs with your family and friends, and coming to a comfortable decision about what you want.

After finding a lump, long delays to start treatment are not advised, but you should not be rushed or pushed into accepting a treatment plan before you are ready, even if it means waiting an extra week or so for surgery to obtain a second opinion or to make up your mind about treatment options. It is best to feel well informed and confident.

Why surgery?

Some women may be completely cured by surgery alone. For others, surgical removal of the tumor is needed because it offers better control of the cancer in the breast than radiation therapy alone. In addition, examination of the tissues removed during surgery provides important information about the type and size of the cancer, the extent of lymph node involvement and the level of estrogen receptors. This information allows the oncologist to determine the stage of the cancer and to tailor any further treatment to your particular case.

For some cancers, surgery is not the best treatment. If the tumor is 'locally advanced,' meaning that there is either a very large breast lump or very enlarged lymph nodes, or it is the inflammatory type of cancer, chemotherapy and radiation may be given first to reduce the size of the tumor. Afterwards, mastectomy may be recommended to further reduce the risk of cancer recurrence in the breast.

In the uncommon situation when the cancer has already spread (metastasized) beyond both the breast and lymph node areas, the initial treatment may include hormones, chemotherapy, radiation and/or Herceptin® rather than surgery.

Choosing a surgeon

How can you find the best surgeon for you? Usually, one surgeon cannot be singled out who is best for everyone in all circumstances. The ideal surgeon is knowledgeable about breast surgery and current practices as well as being skillful in the operating room. Your surgeon should be someone with whom you feel confident.

Many patients are referred to their surgeon through their family doctor. This is fine provided you have confidence in both your family physician and his or her choice. In almost every sizable community there are surgeons who have a special interest in breast cancer. Good information about surgeons can be obtained from women volunteering with the Breast Cancer Visitors program of the Cancer Society or other local support and advocacy groups for breast cancer. You should be able to ask the surgeon questions and get satisfactory answers. If you are not comfortable however, do not be afraid to request a second opinion.

Many cancer centers have breast cancer policy groups. Surgeons participating in such a group will be aware of current trends and practices and may be better able to respond to your questions.

CHAPTER NINETEEN

Types of breast surgery

THERE ARE MANY TYPES OF SURGERY available for the treatment of breast cancer. Why isn't there just one operation? Each procedure has its advantages and disadvantages, depending on the situation. The type of operation best for you depends on a combination of factors: the type of cancer, its size and location, your preference, the surgeon's preference, and the policies of the hospital or cancer center where the treatment takes place.

Take time to consider your options

While it is true that you shouldn't delay surgery too long, most cancers have been present for a number of years and there is no need to rush into the operating room by nightfall. A delay of one to two weeks is usually less important than careful consideration of the surgical options. You should understand your choices and feel comfortable with them. There is time for a well thought out choice based on careful examination of the options, discussions with other patients, a second opinion if desired, and an evaluation of your needs with your family and friends.

It is unwise to assume that you can't understand the details of the treatment and give up control because of feelings of anxiety or fear. Spend a few days talking with others and thinking about which route is best for you. Taking this time to decide what you want leads to an informed choice that ensures that you remain confident and have some measure of control. In the long run, this is time well spent.

Operations that save the breast

Partial mastectomy: removing a small amount of the breast

A partial mastectomy (also known as 'lumpectomy,' 'segmental mastectomy' or 'wide excision') is an operation that removes the cancer plus some surrounding normal breast tissue (Figure 18). This has become the most commonly performed surgery for the treatment of breast cancer. Studies have found that a partial mastectomy followed by radiation gives a woman the same chance of survival and control of the cancer as does an operation that removes the whole breast.

When the cancer and breast tissue is taken out, careful attention is paid to the edges of the tissue being removed to make certain that they don't contain any cancer. The objective is to remove the cancer lump along with any of the 'tentacles' that extend into the normal breast tissue while still leaving enough tissue so that the breast looks cosmetically 'normal.'

After a skillfully done partial mastectomy for a small tumor, the breast should look similar to the untreated breast (Figure 19). The size of the area removed depends partly on the location of the tumor and the size of the breast. The goal of the surgery is to remove the cancer but leave the breast as normal-appearing as possible. Ask your surgeon how much normal tissue will be removed. In general, removal of more than 1.0 to 1.5 cm of tissue beyond the cancer itself is rarely required. However, it is not always possible to know the exact extent of the cancer in the breast before the operation. Removal of an excessive amount of normal tissue will adversely affect the way your breast will look after surgery.

Partial mastectomy combined with axillary dissection (removal of lymph nodes in the armpit)

Along with removing the actual tumor from the breast, lymph nodes are usually removed from the armpit. This is known as an axillary dissection, and may be done at the same time as a partial mastectomy. There are two reasons for doing this. Axillary dissection

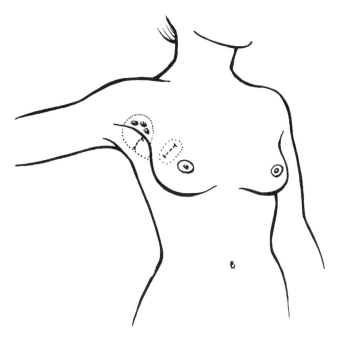

Figure 18: A partial mastectomy involves removing some normal breast tissue surrounding the cancer. The axillary dissection is performed through a separate incision in the armpit.

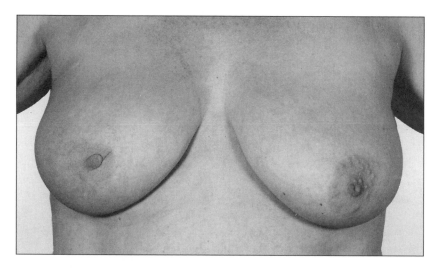

Figure 19: Five years after a partial mastectomy and radiotherapy for a cancer of the right breast.

removes any of the cancer that may have spread to the lymph nodes and by analyzing the lymph nodes under the microscope, the pathologist can determine whether the cancer has spread to these nodes. This will help determine the type of chemotherapy, radiation or hormone therapy that is offered after surgery.

The axilla is divided into three levels and usually the first two levels of lymph nodes are removed in the axillary dissection. A properly performed axillary dissection will usually contain more than 10 lymph nodes, although this number is variable. The deepest lymph nodes, which are found just below the collar bone (level 3 nodes) are usually not removed unless they appear to be diseased.

An axillary dissection is usually done under general anesthetic and may require a night in hospital. A separate incision is made in the armpit (Figure 18). Just before closing the wound, the surgeon places a small tube, called a 'drain,' into the area where the lymph nodes were, to collect fluid that would otherwise accumulate. The other end of the tube comes out through the skin and is sewn in place. In a few days, when less fluid is draining through the tube, the drain is removed.

Sentinel node biopsy

A new technique has been developed to try to eliminate the need to remove lymph nodes that do not contain cancer. This technique involves 'labeling' axillary nodes closest to the cancer. A blue dye and/or a radioactive agent is injected around the cancer or biopsy cavity in the breast. Sometimes the tracer is just injected into the breast below the areola. The dye or radioactive tracer is absorbed into the lymphatic channels and travels to the first few lymph nodes 'upstream' from the cancer. A small incision is made over the labeled node(s) and the one or two 'sentinel' nodes are removed and examined to see if there is any cancer involvement.

One problem with the procedure, though, is that getting accurate information from the sentinel node biopsy requires considerable expertise on the part of the surgeon, and close integration between the surgeon, the nuclear medicine department and the pathologist. Even in expert hands, approximately 10% of patients with cancer in the axilla will not have this found by a sentinel node biopsy. This "false negative" rate is higher for surgeons who are just learning the sentinel node biopsy technique. It is recommended that surgeons not stop doing full axillary dissections until they have personally done at least 30 sentinel node procedures successfully and proven that their 'false negative' rate is less than 10%.

Sentinel node biopsy alone is not a procedure that can produce accurate results when done on an intermittent or occasional basis. Sentinel node biopsy is most useful for solitary breast cancers less than 5 cm diameter when there are no nodes felt in the axilla (armpit). If there are multiple cancers in one breast or the cancer is locally advanced (large or invading the skin or muscles) or there are enlarged, suspicious nodes in the axilla, the sentinel node biopsy should not be done.

Operations that remove the breast

Total (simple) mastectomy

A total mastectomy is the removal of the entire breast and nipple without removing any muscles or axillary lymph nodes. This procedure is useful if the entire breast must be removed and there is no suspicion of cancer in the axillary nodes. For example, if a woman who has a strong family history of breast cancer decides to have both breasts removed to eliminate the risk of developing breast cancer (not a decision to be taken lightly), a total mastectomy is the best operation because it removes all of the breast tissue while preserving the normal lymph nodes and muscle.

Modified-radical mastectomy

Modified radical mastectomy was the standard surgical procedure for breast cancer for many years. It involves the total removal of the breast along with the axillary lymph nodes, some skin and the nipple (Figure 20). It is called 'modified' because it does not remove the chest wall muscles or nerves and removes fewer lymph nodes than the original radical mastectomy (see below). A modified radical mastectomy is suitable for most patients with early stage breast cancer who are not interested in conserving their breasts.

An incision is made over the breast. The resulting scar, after removal of the breast and lymph nodes, is long and straight or diagonal across the chest wall (Figure 20). Ask your surgeon how the scar will look and what measures he or she can take to make it easier for you to consider reconstructive surgery if you decide to

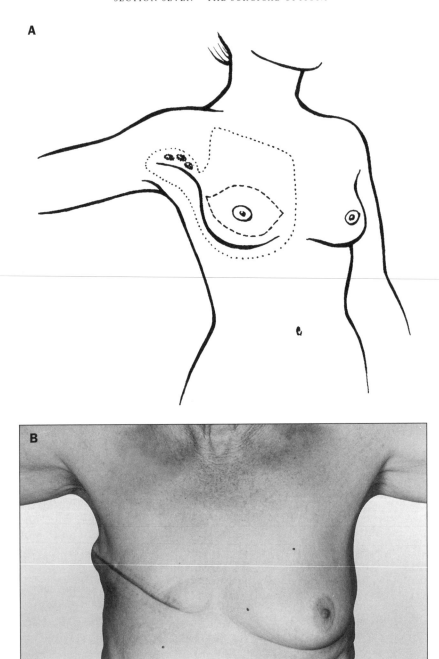

Figure 20: Extent of tissue removed (A) and appearance after a modified radical mastectomy (B).

have it later. A modified radical mastectomy is usually done under general anesthetic and often requires a night in hospital The armpit lymph nodes are removed and a drain tube is left in place to avoid fluid build-up.

Radical mastectomy

Radical mastectomy includes removal of the breast, the pectoralis major and minor chest wall muscles, some nerves, the nipple, the skin, and all of the lymph nodes in the armpit right up to the collarbone. The incision goes all the way from the armpit down to the top of the abdomen. The chest wall ends up looking deformed due to the loss of muscle. Because so much tissue is removed a skin graft is often needed. These days a radical mastectomy should rarely be necessary.

Subcutaneous mastectomy

As with the simple mastectomy, this operation has been used by some to prevent future cancer in a woman at high risk. In a subcutaneous mastectomy, the breast tissue is 'dug out' through a small incision while preserving the breast, skin and nipple. The main disadvantage of this operation is that approximately 15% of the breast glandular tissue is left behind. Therefore it is an unsuitable operation for complete cancer prevention. In addition, results of reconstructive surgery may not be quite as good after a subcutaneous mastectomy.

Mastectomy and immediate reconstruction

Many women who need or desire a mastectomy (Chapter 20) may also be interested in reconstruction (Chapter 34). It may be possible to perform the reconstruction at the same time as the mastectomy (called immediate reconstruction). The potential for reconstruction or immediate reconstruction should be discussed prior to mastectomy.

CHAPTER TWENTY

What type of surgery is best for me?

Does one type of surgery offer a better chance of cure?

THE AIM OF SURGERY IS TO GIVE you the best chance of being cured of cancer. Usually, the choice is between a partial mastectomy with an axillary dissection (or sentinel node biopsy) and a modified radical mastectomy (differences explained in Chapter 19). Studies have shown that partial mastectomy and axillary dissection followed by radiation and a modified radical mastectomy without radiation provide an equal chance of cure and a high chance (85% to 95%) of controlling the cancer in the breast or chest wall. Therefore, your choice of one operation or the other need NOT be based on the 'relapse rate.'

How do I choose the right surgery?

A partial mastectomy is suitable for about 75% of patients. Usually a woman will feel better about herself if she can keep her breast, but there are a number of other factors you and your surgeon should consider:
- Your preference
- The surgical issues, including the size of the breast, size of the tumor, its location and the type of cancer cells
- Your age and general health

- Your ability to undergo radiation
- Your availability for regular follow-up visits after the surgery is done.

Your preference counts

Whenever possible, YOUR PREFERENCE should be the deciding factor. A total mastectomy may seem like the better solution for a woman whose breasts are difficult to examine or who is 'never going to trust that breast again'. On the other hand, a partial mastectomy conserves the breast and avoids the discomfort and necessity of wearing an artificial breast (prosthesis). The main disadvantages of a partial mastectomy are the inconvenience and side-effects of several weeks of daily radiation treatments that are usually required after a breast-saving operation (see Chapters 24 to 26).

Studies have shown that in the years after surgery, women have similar levels of distress regardless of whether they have had their breast removed or saved. In other words, the diagnosis of cancer causes anxiety no matter what type of surgery is done. Other studies have shown that women who are given the choice of surgical treatment feel empowered and therefore adjust to the diagnosis of breast cancer more easily than women who are told to have a particular type of operation.

Surgical issues

Surgical considerations include the size and location of the tumor compared to the size of the breast. If the tumor is large and the breast is small, a partial mastectomy may remove too much breast tissue, leaving a disappointing cosmetic result. In general, tumors larger than 5 cm are better treated by a modified radical mastectomy, with the option of breast reconstruction either later or at the same time. As a rule, tumors that are smaller than 3 cm can almost always be removed by a partial mastectomy. The size of the breast must be carefully considered for tumors between 3 and 5 cm. If the tumor is very large, it may be advisable to have chemotherapy and radiation before the surgery. If the tumor shrinks dramatically, it could still be possible to conserve the breast.

The location of the tumor can also affect the cosmetic result of a partial mastectomy. If the tumor is in the center of the breast the nipple may have to be removed, resulting in a less satisfactory appearance as well as loss of nipple sensation. If the partial mastectomy is done well, however, the result may be superior to a mastectomy and reconstruction, or mastectomy and a prosthesis.

About 1% of women are found to have two or more tumors in one breast. If there are multiple tumors within the breast, it might not be possible to remove all the affected areas without removing the whole breast. Multiple tumors are usually identified before surgery on the mammograms, but sometimes they are only identified in the pathology report after surgery. If a mastectomy is felt to be the best choice, it may be possible to do an immediate breast reconstruction during the same anesthetic (see Chapter 34).

Your overall health affects your ability to undergo radiation

The state of your general health is an important factor when deciding if a partial mastectomy is the best treatment for you. Since radiation is generally required after a partial mastectomy, this type of operation should not be recommended if you are not suitable for radiation. Radiation treatment may be difficult for someone who is elderly or very weak and has difficulty visiting a clinic every day for three to six weeks. Patients who cannot lie flat on the treatment table, or who cannot lift their arms over their head for the radiation treatment (for example after a stroke) will have difficulty with this part of the treatment. Therefore, they may be advised to have a modified radical mastectomy instead.

You would also be considered unsuitable for radiation treatment if it is felt that you have a high risk of severe side effects (see Chapter 26). Some women who have certain medical conditions should not receive radiation if they have a choice. These conditions include severe lung disease, or heart disease. Women with systemic lupus erythematosus (SLE), scleroderma or ataxia-telangiectasia could have severe reactions and scarring from the radiation so they are probably best treated by a modified radical mastectomy. Women who are pregnant should also avoid radiation because of possible harm to the fetus.

Women with very large breasts tend to get more radiation side effects because of the large amount of tissue that must be treated.

Also, radiation should not be given to a woman who has already received therapeutic doses of radiation to the same breast in the past.

Partial mastectomy means regular follow-up visits

After a partial mastectomy and radiation, the breast should be carefully observed on a regular basis to detect any early, potentially curable cancer recurrence. You should get to know the 'normal feel' of your treated breast. After surgery and radiation there are often areas of thickening or lumpiness. This is normal but report changes in the lumpiness to your doctor. The best way to monitor your breasts is by a monthly breast self-examination. You should also have a physical examination every six to 12 months done by a physician with experience in the follow-up of women after partial mastectomy and radiation.

A mammogram six months after the radiation treatment is completed may be recommended, followed by mammograms of both breasts annually. It is important that all women with breast cancer realize they should have regular mammograms unless both breasts have been removed.

Is a partial mastectomy and axillary dissection better than a modified radical mastectomy?

In most cases, a breast-saving operation such as a partial mastectomy with an axillary dissection (or sentinel node biopsy) followed by radiation provides an equal chance of cure and control of the disease as a modified radical mastectomy. This doesn't mean that a partial mastectomy is better, but it does allow you to make a choice. You should consider the risks and benefits of both, and your doctors should give you sufficient information and the respect to allow you to make an informed choice. Studies have shown that when offered a choice, about 75% to 85% of women elect to have a breast saving operation.

The advantage of a breast-saving operation is that the breast is saved! This must be weighed against the need for a series of radiation treatments. The advantages of a modified radical mastectomy are that the treatment is over at once and radiation treatments can be avoided in most cases. Also, if there is a large cancer or more than one cancer in the affected breast, or if certain conditions make radiation more hazardous, modified radical mastectomy may be the better option. A mastectomy means that the breast is removed completely. Since each person is unique, it is appropriate and healthy for you to participate in this crucial decision.

Six international scientific studies have compared breast-saving operations to modified radical mastectomy. These have shown that a partial mastectomy followed by radiation therapy to the breast provides an equal chance of survival compared to modified radical mastectomy. Some authorities feel that breast conservation plus radiation therapy is preferable, since it achieves equal survival, and provides sexual and psychological advantages.

CHAPTER TWENTY-ONE

Hospitalization and recovering from surgery

Dealing with hospitalization

YOU MAY FIND THE HOSPITAL'S ADMISSION routine a source of frustration. Some patients feel that they are answering the same questions over and over again and wonder why nobody seems to be listening. Hospital procedures require that a patient be admitted by the clerk, the ward nurse and a number of doctors, including the surgeon and anesthetist. In a teaching hospital the list may also include a student nurse, a medical student, an intern and a resident. Be patient. They are listening, but each of them requires slightly different information. Also, the many questions ensure that everyone knows you individually and that any allergies you suffer and medications that you take regularly are recorded.

The recovery room

In the recovery room nurses carefully monitor you as you wake up. Often, patients are confused for a short period. Also, you may have a sore throat. This is a temporary discomfort caused by the breathing tube that was used to help you breathe during the operation. The doctor will have provided a list of orders, including pain relief and other medications. You may feel nauseated from the anesthetic or get shivers when you wake up.

Your surgeon might come to talk to you here, although you may be too groggy to remember much. Only a few preliminary findings will be known right away. The full pathology report is usually not available for three to five days.

Notifying your significant other

There is usually someone you will want the surgeon to contact when the operation is finished, so that person's name and phone number should be clearly written in your chart. If your significant other is waiting in the hospital, make sure it is clear exactly where they are since the surgeon may want to talk to them while you are in the recovery room.

The ward

The type of operation and your recovery time will determine how long you stay in hospital. Most patients go home the same day if the operation involved only the breast and the next day if surgery involved both the breast and the axilla (armpit). The sooner patients start moving around after surgery the fewer problems they have, so you will be urged to get out of bed and walk up and down the halls.

Pain

After the surgery there will be some pain that can be controlled with pain killers. Everyone is different, so let the nurse know when you are in pain so you can receive medication according to your needs. Many pain killers can cause nausea and constipation but this is generally mild and temporary.

Drains

If you have an axillary dissection or a modified radical mastectomy, you may have one or two drains in the area for the first few days to prevent fluid accumulation. The drains are usually checked and removed by a home care nurse several days after you leave hospital. Sometimes, after the drain is removed the fluid builds up again causing a tender swelling in the armpit. This is called a seroma. The seroma may need to be drained using a syringe. This can be done easily in the surgeon's office during an outpatient visit.

Sutures

Some stitches (sutures) may eventually dissolve on their own while other, non-absorbable sutures or staples need to be removed, usually a week to ten days after the surgery. Ask your surgeon what sort of sutures will be used. The redness of your scar will gradually fade over several months.

Going home: ask questions before you leave

You are bound to have questions about what you can do when you get home, so write them down and be prepared to rattle off the list when you see your doctor after the surgery. Make sure you have a clear understanding about what you can and cannot do, what exercises you should do to start moving your arm, when to start them (Chapter 33), when you should see the surgeon again and when you will be referred to a medical or radiation oncologist. Also, be sure to have a prescription for pain killers because you may need them, especially as you get more active.

Most women suffer some pain along the incision and under the arm that lasts from several days to a few weeks or longer. This can be controlled with pain medications. Later on, some women complain of a tightness or discomfort over the chest area which, although mild, is often bothersome and longer-lasting. This may be helped by physiotherapy (see Chapter 33). The incision usually heals within a few weeks, but can take somewhat longer in women who have had radiation before surgery.

The risk of infection with breast surgery is usually low, but if there is a foul-smelling drainage, increasingly red and tender skin or any fever, there may be an infection and it should be treated promptly with antibiotics.

With any surgery, there is a risk of bleeding afterwards, even though the surgeon has been extremely careful. This can result in a hematoma (blood clot in the tissues) which can be swollen, painful and leave the breast bruised-looking. Usually, the hematoma subsides on its own, but if it is large, it may need to be drained.

After breast surgery many women complain about numbness in the back of the underarm or on the chest wall. This is usually due to nerves being cut or stretched during the operation and may improve in the months ahead.

Breast surgery is emotionally difficult for many women. Often, it is difficult for a patient to look at her own body, let alone show her spouse, friends or family the scars. As the incision fades and you use your arm, you can begin to heal. A breast cancer support group and a physiotherapy consultation are often helpful to regain a positive sense of your body.

A note about visitors

A stay in hospital tends to bring friends and relatives out of the woodwork. Depending on your personality, this may or may not please you. If the visiting is too tiring, speak to your nurse and visitors can be restricted. Seeing people and discussing the situation can be helpful, especially with supportive people who are close to you, but do not let the socializing wear you out.

Obtaining a breast prosthesis

If you have been treated with a mastectomy, you may want to consider a prosthesis or breast reconstruction (see Chapter 34). The prosthesis is a soft, somewhat heavy plastic form that comes in many shapes and sizes to match the many shapes and sizes of women's breasts.

Breast Cancer Visitor volunteers from the Cancer Society will often supply a soft, 'fluffy' breast form of cotton that you can wear temporarily in your own bra. This helps fill out your clothes but does not have the weight or shape of your other breast. A fitted prosthesis will help you feel better and walk straighter. Once the initial pain and swelling of the mastectomy has settled and the wound is healed, you are ready for a 'fitting.' This is often four to six weeks after surgery.

Breast prostheses are not one-size-fits-all and just picking a form off the shelf will not give you the best fit. You need to consider the size, shape and weight of your remaining breast to get a good match. The traditional prosthesis is sold with a specially designed bra with a pocket into which the prosthesis can fit. A recent innovation is a prosthesis which directly adheres to the chest wall. It is attached to the chest by strips of velcro which are glued to the chest and the underside of the prosthesis. Body heat activates the adhesive properties of the glue and the velcro strips remain on the chest wall for a week to 10 days. They come off without the tearing or sting of usual adhesive plasters.

Additional garments are available such as bathing suits and nightgowns that are specially designed to hold the prosthesis.

Depending on where you live, there may be many or just a few places to buy a prosthesis such as department or drug stores. In larger towns you can find stores that specialize in selling and fitting prostheses and garments to wear with the prosthesis. Your surgeon, support group, local Cancer Society office or nurses at your cancer center should be able to direct you to a store. Breast prostheses are a medical appliance so you should check if the cost is covered by your medical insurance.

Preventing recurrence of cancer

Additional treatment following surgery: Radiation, chemotherapy and hormone treatment

Why is additional treatment needed?

EVEN WHEN THE CANCER APPEARS to have been totally removed, the surgeon can never be sure that he or she 'got it all'. This is because microscopic cells may be in the remaining skin, breast tissue or lymph nodes, or cancer cells may have spread elsewhere in the body as tiny, undetectable metastases. This is a frustrating problem because only time will tell whether or not the operation was indeed a cure.

Because of this, treatment is given in addition to surgery, as a preventive measure, in case cancer is still present. This preventive treatment given in addition to surgery is called 'adjuvant' therapy, and is a normal part of breast cancer treatment for the majority of women. The treatments used for adjuvant therapy include radiation, chemotherapy Herceptin® and hormonal agents.

Who should receive adjuvant therapy?

Because we are not able to detect the presence of just a few microscopic cancer cells, each patient's risk of cancer recurrence is assessed based on the surgical findings and the pathology report (see Table 4).

Based on this assessment, adjuvant therapy may or may not be recommended to a particular patient. For instance, a woman with a very low risk of cancer recurrence and a high probability (more than 95%) of being cured by surgery alone may not require any adjuvant therapy. New recommendations are constantly being developed to keep pace with the ever-improving understanding of breast cancer. Still, most women do receive some form of adjuvant therapy today.

When should adjuvant therapy start?

Adjuvant therapy is usually started within four to twelve weeks after surgery. It is sometimes difficult to accept the need for additional treatment so soon, especially because it requires one to admit the possibility of the cancer returning. Ideally, the concept of adjuvant therapy will have been discussed before surgery to give you more time to consider it and come to terms with the reasons for it.

Types of adjuvant therapy

Radiotherapy

Adjuvant radiotherapy is almost always given after partial mastectomy. Although the cancer may seem to have been removed completely, the likelihood of the cancer coming back in the same breast may be relatively high (10% to 40% over 10 years without radiation). Radiation to the breast can significantly reduce this risk.

Women who have had their breast removed may also be treated by adjuvant radiation if the tumor was large (more than 5 cm), if it was invading the skin or chest wall, or if several (more than 25% for instance) of the lymph nodes were cancerous. In this situation, adjuvant radiation decreases the chance of the cancer recurring on the chest wall or in the lymph node areas, and may improve survival (see Chapter 25).

Chemotherapy

Chemotherapy is the use of drugs given orally, or more often, directly into the vein (see Chapters 27 to 29). Adjuvant chemotherapy is given after surgery when there is a risk of residual cancer cells re-growing as metastases throughout the body. Adjuvant chemotherapy decreases the risk of this recurrence and therefore increases the number of women cured.

Hormone therapy

Hormone therapy is usually given as pills and can be effective against breast cancer cells that may have 'escaped.' Hormone therapy blocks the effect of estrogen on the tumor or reduces the level of estrogen in the blood. (The connection between estrogen and cancer growth is discussed in Chapter 30.) Hormone therapy is only effective if the tumor is sensitive to hormone stimulation (estrogen receptor or progesterone receptor positive) and is used in both pre and post menoposal women. In premenopausal women, ovaries are the primary source of estrogen. Surgical removal of the ovaries or an injection to stop ovarian function may be recommended.

Herceptin® therapy

Herceptin® (transtuzamab) is given as an intravenous injection every three weeks for a year or sometimes longer. Herceptin® has recently been shown to decrease the risk of recurrence and death for the 20% to 25% of women whose breast cancer overexpresses the HER2 gene. It has no benefit if the woman's tumor does not overexpress HER2.

Combined adjuvant therapy

Depending on the type of surgery and the extent of the cancer when it is discovered, more than one type of adjuvant therapy may be offered. Each woman's situation is different. Therefore, one woman may receive both radiotherapy and hormone therapy following her surgery, while another may get chemotherapy alone. When more than one type of adjuvant therapy is used, it is called 'combined modality treatment.'

CHAPTER TWENTY-THREE

Treatment of in situ breast cancer

Treatment of ductal carcinoma in situ

DUCTAL CARCINOMA IN SITU (DCIS) refers to breast cancer that is still entirely within the milk ducts of the breast and has not invaded nearby tissues. Therefore, it has not had any chance to spread to other parts of the body. Chapter 13 provides a description of this type of cancer. DCIS is being diagnosed much more frequently today because of the increasing number of women having regular mammograms. In some individuals, DCIS might never progress to form an invasive cancer and might never be a threat to a woman's life. However, if left untreated, some cases of DCIS will become invasive and spread to other parts of the body.

The goal of treatment of DCIS is to completely remove or control the cancer cells before they form an invasive cancer. If a breast-saving procedure is used, the aim of treatment is to have less than a 5% risk of recurrence in the breast during the first 10 years after surgery.

Breast conservation is an option

In the past, the traditional treatment for ductal carcinoma in situ was a simple (total) mastectomy to prevent the progression to invasive cancer. The cure rate after such a mastectomy is close to 100%. Mastectomy remains an acceptable treatment for DCIS.

However, many women are interested in a treatment that conserves the breast and still provides an excellent chance for cure.

Studies have shown that radiation therapy to the breast after a partial mastectomy can significantly reduce the risk of recurrent cancer in the breast. For women who want to save their breast, partial mastectomy plus radiation is considered the standard treatment.

To remove the entire ductal carcinoma in situ and conserve the breast, it is critical that the surgeon plan the operation with a clear idea of the mammogram appearance of the cancer. As well, the pathologist must systematically inspect many samples of the removed tissue to ensure that no invasive cancer is present and to give an estimate of how complete the excision is.

In most cases, even if the in situ cancer appears to have been completely removed, radiation therapy is given. Together, the surgery and radiation provide a greater than 90% chance of local control of the cancer. If recurrence in the breast does develop, most cases will be cured with a mastectomy. Therefore, with careful attention to the type and extent of DCIS, and the use of partial mastectomy plus radiation therapy, approximately 90% of women can save their breasts; and, the ultimate cure rate is equal to women who have a total mastectomy.

The woman who chooses breast conservation requires lifelong follow-up so that if recurrence develops, she can receive treatment at a stage when a cure is still possible. About half of the recurrences in the breast will be DCIS and the rest will be invasive. Usually, if the recurrence occurs after excision and radiation therapy for the initial cancer, a total mastectomy is necessary.

If the ductal carcinoma in situ is extensive

If the in situ cancer is widespread (more than 5 cm across or involving more than 1/4 of the breast), the amount of tissue that must be removed often leads to unacceptable disfigurement of the breast. Also, even after radiation therapy there may be a high (30% to 40%) chance of recurrence in the breast. Since about half of these recurrences will be invasive, with the possibility of distant spread, when the in situ cancer is very extensive, total mastectomy with or without reconstruction is usually recommended to maximize the chances of a long-term cure.

Wide excision alone for very small DCIS

For some women with relatively small areas of DCIS, it may be possible to save the breast and avoid radiation therapy. For this procedure to be successful, the cancer should be less than 2 cm in diameter on both the mammogram and pathology, AND the cancer should not be the high-grade subtype (very abnormal-looking cells with necrosis) AND to be confidant that the DCIS has been completely removed, there should be at least 1 cm of normal breast tissue between any ducts containing DCIS and the edge of the excision specimen. Radiation therapy may still reduce the risk of breast recurrence further, but because the risk is quite low with surgery alone in these cases, only a few women among every hundred treated would benefit. Research in this area is ongoing.

High-grade ductal carcinoma in situ

Ductal carcinoma in situ that has very abnormal-appearing cells (grade 3; see Chapter 14) and a lot of necrosis in the milk ducts tends to develop recurrences more often than the other types of in situ cancer and also tends to form invasive cancers earlier. These types of lesions are sometimes called 'comedocarcinoma'. To achieve the best control, some authorities recommend adding radiation after wide excision for any size of comedocarcinoma, even if it is very small.

The boxed information at the end of this chapter summarizes recommendations for the management of ductal carcinoma in situ.

Tamoxifen and other hormonal therapy

Tamoxifen, at a dose of 20 mg per day for five years, can decrease both the recurrence of in situ cancer and the development of invasive breast cancer in women with in situ disease. Tamoxifen may be particularly helpful if the DCIS was estrogen receptor positive. Tamoxifen may also decrease the chance of developing cancer in the opposite breast. However, studies to date suggest that overall survival, 10 years after the initial diagnosis and treatment of a DCIS was equal, whether women received tamoxifen or not.

Tamoxifen may cause side effects, including hot flashes, mood disturbance (depression), a small risk of endometrial cancer and an increased risk of thrombosis (blood clots). Therefore, although women with DCIS may benefit from tamoxifen, each woman's risk of side effects should be balanced against the risk of cancer recurrence before making a decision about taking the drug. Women who have had bilateral mastectomies (both breasts removed) and are not at risk of further local disease, or have a history of blood clots, or have other severe health problems or advanced age and are unlikely to live another 10 years, will not benefit sufficiently from tamoxifen to outweigh the side effects.

In recent years there have been several studies that have shown that aromatase inhibitors (see Chapter 30) used on their own or following several years of tamoxifen, have a greater ability to reduce breast cancer recurrence compared to using tamoxifen alone. All those studies involved patients with invasive breast cancer. Current studies are examining the role of aromatase inhibitors in postmenopausal women with DCIS and as a breast cancer prevention agent. At the present time however, aromatase inhibitors are not recommended as treatment for patients with DCIS.

Treatment of lobular carcinoma in situ

Women with lobular carcinoma in situ (also called lobular neoplasia) have a higher than average risk of developing an invasive breast cancer some time in the future. Overall, the chance of developing breast cancer is about 20% to 30% over the next 20 years. The risk of developing invasive breast cancer is related to the extent of lobular carcinoma in situ in the breast biopsy. If there are just focal ('local') deposits, the risk is not much higher than for an 'average' woman of the same age. If the lobular carcinoma in situ is very extensive, the risk of subsequent cancer may be from four to 10 times higher than for an 'average' woman. The invasive cancers are about as likely to develop in either breast, so any therapy has to be directed at both breasts.

One course of action is to undertake careful, regular screening and follow-up. Another, drastic choice that has been used is preventive removal of both breasts (bilateral 'prophylactic' mastectomy; see Chapter 19 on 'total mastectomy'). This is only done on rare occasions when a woman's fear of developing breast cancer outweighs her desire to save her breasts. This surgery may be recommended if a woman with lobular carcinoma in situ has a strong family history of breast cancer.

Lobular cancers are almost always estrogen receptor-positive (see Chapter 30), which suggests that the anti-estrogen drug tamoxifen might be able to 'block' the stimulating effect of natural estrogens and help prevent the development of invasive cancers. A large study demonstrated that for women with lobular carcinoma in situ, tamoxifen can reduce the chance of developing an invasive breast cancer. Although tamoxifen is usually well tolerated, it does have some potentially serious side effects such as blood clots in the legs and lungs and a higher risk of developing cancer of the endometrium (uterus). In addition, tamoxifen can affect one's quality of life by causing hot flashes, vaginal dryness and/or depression.

Because of the potential serious side effects, it is not clear-cut whether all women with lobular carcinoma in situ should take tamoxifen to prevent the development of breast cancer. Each woman needs to consider other options as well as take into account her individual likelihood of developing invasive cancer (age, family history, extensiveness of the lobular carcinoma in situ) and her general health (tamoxifen cannot be taken if she has had phlebitis or blood clots in the past). Women with a family history of breast cancer, extensive lobular carcinoma in situ and no history of phlebitis may benefit sufficiently from tamoxifen to warrant taking it for five years.

Options for treatment of the breast with DCIS

Wide excision (partial mastectomy) alone is appropriate if:
- The cancer is less than 2 cm AND
- Not a high grade subtype AND
- A good margin (≥ 1 cm) of normal breast tissue was seen between the cancer and the edge of the surgical specimen

Wide excision (partial mastectomy) plus radiation therapy is appropriate if:
- The cancer is less than 5 cm in diameter OR
- Was the grade 3 subtype OR
- The margin between the DCIS and the edge of the removed tissue is <1 cm
- An option for any size or type of DCIS

Simple (total) mastectomy is appropriate if:
- The cancer is extensive (more than 5 cm in diameter on pathology or width of calcifications on mammogram) OR
- The margins still show cancer after two attempts at wide excision OR
- The patient chooses this option for any size or type of in situ cancer

---

SECTION NINE

Radiation therapy

CHAPTER TWENTY-FOUR

Radiation therapy: What is it?

How does radiation work?

RADIATION THERAPY, ALSO CALLED 'RADIOTHERAPY,' is the use of high-energy rays to kill cancer cells. Radiation works by damaging the cells so that they eventually die. Since radiation will damage any type of cell, either normal or cancerous, that lies in the path of the beam, great care must be taken to aim the beam only at the required tissue and avoid healthy tissue as much as possible.

Fortunately, normal cells repair themselves from radiation damage more completely than cancer cells do. So, by giving the radiation in a series of small treatments, usually once a day, normal cells have a chance to recover between treatments while the cancer cells die.

When is radiation given?

Radiation therapy is used to help prevent recurrence or progression of cancer in one specific part of the body, for example the breast, chest wall or lymph nodes. After a lumpectomy, radiation is directed at the breast to kill any possible 'leftover' cancer cells. It may also be used to treat metastatic cancer in a particular place in the body. For instance, if breast cancer has spread to a woman's hip bone and causes pain, radiation to the hip will kill the cancer cells there and relieve the pain.

The benefits and side effects of radiation therapy are generally restricted to the area being treated. In contrast, chemotherapy agents, Herceptin® and hormones are absorbed into the blood stream and affect many parts of the body.

The procedure for getting radiotherapy

The process can be considered in three steps:
1. Deciding whether treatment is advisable.
2. Attending a 'planning' visit to the radiation department where the area of treatment will be identified, marked and measurements will be taken to calculate the radiation dose.
3. Receiving radiotherapy during daily visits according to a planned schedule.

The treatment decision

You make the decision to proceed with radiotherapy in consultation with a radiation oncologist (a specialist in radiation therapy). The issues to consider are described in Chapter 26.

The planning session

The purpose of this session is to plan exactly how the x-ray machine is to be directed, given your individual size and body shape, and the part of the body that requires treatment.

The area to be treated can be marked out by eye or by using a machine called a 'simulator.' The simulator sends low-energy x-rays through the body onto a screen or film so that the target area to be treated can be determined exactly. Very specific information is recorded during the planning session so that the treatment machine can be accurately positioned each day. Frequently today, a CT-simulator is used. The CT is a large, donut-shaped machine. The patient lies on a table and is moved through the 'donut' while x-rays are taken. The CT produces a cross-sectional image of the breast and internal anatomy of the chest (Figure 21). The CT makes it easier for the radiation oncologist to design a treatment plan that excludes from the radiation beam as much heart and lung as possible.

Two to four permanent ink dots, the size of a small freckle, are often placed at the center or corner of the treatment area. These 'tattoos' are reference points used for the daily treatments and can

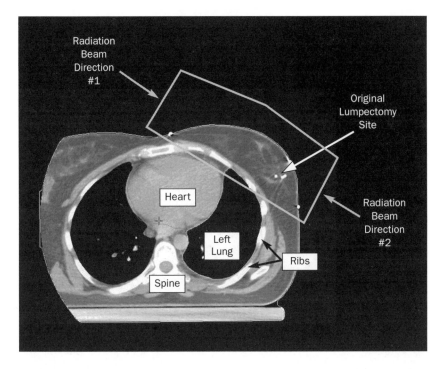

Figure 21: A radiation-planning CT Scan through the breast showing the organs nearby that are at risk of side effects from radiation, the lungs, heart, ribs and skin. The original lumpectomy site in the left breast is marked with a dashed arrow. Radiation is directed through the breast from side to side and is angled to avoid as much lung and heart tissue as possible.

be useful if radiation is being considered again sometime in the future. Sometimes temporary ink marks are also placed on the skin to help with daily treatment set ups.

Treatment sessions

The amount of radiation you receive and number of daily visits depends on the amount of tissue to be treated, and whether the goal of treatment is to treat a mass of cancer, prevent a recurrence after surgery or to relieve symptoms. Usually, adjuvant or curative radiation requires from three to six weeks of daily treatments. When the goal is symptom relief, a single treatment or one to three weeks of treatment is usually sufficient.

What happens during radiation treatment?

Radiation treatments are painless. In fact, when the machine is on, the only thing you'll notice is a slight whirring sound. Treatments may be given from several angles each day (Figure 22).

You will be in the treatment room for about 10 to 20 minutes. Most of this time is spent carefully adjusting the treatment machine, called a linear accelerator, so that it is positioned correctly. During a typical radiation treatment session the machine is turned on for only one to three minutes per treated area each day.

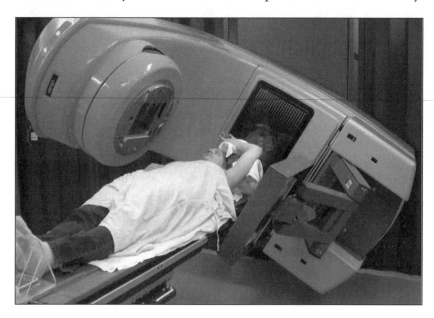

Figure 22: Woman getting ready for treatment on a radiotherapy machine.

How much radiation is given during radiotherapy?

The amount of radiation given is limited by the amount the normal tissues can tolerate. The basic unit of radiation dose is called a Gray. The amount of radiation received during a chest x-ray is approximately 0.005 Gray. For a mammogram it is 0.003 Gray. In contrast, the typical total dose used to treat the whole breast during cancer therapy ranges from 40 Gray (divided into 15 daily doses given over three weeks) up to 50 Gray (divided into 25 daily doses given over five weeks). If only a part of the breast is being treated (see Chapter 25), the dose of radiation varies considerably with the partial breast radiation technique that is used and whether it is done as a single treatment during the lumpectomy or as a week of treatment after surgery.

Brachytherapy—another way to give radiation

In this procedure, instead of using a machine that sends out an x-ray beam, a tiny piece of radioactive material is implanted directly into a tumor or into the area where from which the tumor was removed. Radioactive iridium is the substance most often used for brachytherapy, but other materials such as radioactive gold or palladium are also used.

Under local or general anesthetic, hollow tubes are placed into the breast around the surgical site. These are stitched into place. This is called the 'implant.' Later, in the clinic, the doctor or technician places the radioactive material into the tubes, usually with a remote-control device. Treatments may be given twice a day for a week. The patient has the tubes in her breast for the week but she is not radioactive when she goes home.

Depending on the radioactive material used and the dose, the radiation sources may be left in place continuously or may be inserted into the implant tubes once or twice a day for several days. During active treatment, the hospital room is considered to be radioactive and visitors are restricted.

Very recently, an experimental form of brachytherapy has been described using a permanent implant. In this technique, several dozen radioactive pellets the size of an uncooked grain of rice, are inserted into the breast tissue surrounding the lumpectomy site. These radioactive 'seeds' are left in the breast permanently. The side-effects and benefits of this technique are being tested in a research study involving women with very small tumors that appear to have been completely removed and who do not have any cancer spread to the axilla (armpit) lymph nodes.

Can radiation be repeated at some time in the future?

When giving radiotherapy to a part of the body, the idea is to maximize the destruction of the cancer while staying within safe limits on normal surrounding tissues. Therefore a part has been given maximum radiation at some time in the past, treatment of that area must not be repeated. Occasionally, however, if a fairly low dose of radiation was used and cancer re-growth causes symptoms at the same site, the area can be re-treated. If an entirely new area of the body develops problems from cancer, it can be considered for radiation treatment.

CHAPTER TWENTY-FIVE

Who benefits from radiation therapy?

THERE ARE FOUR GENERAL SITUATIONS in which radiotherapy is used for women with breast cancer:

- after a breast-saving partial mastectomy
- after a modified radical mastectomy when there is a high chance of recurrence on the chest wall or in the lymph nodes
- as treatment for locally advanced cancer when surgery is not advisable
- for the relief of symptoms due to cancer recurrence on the chest wall or metastases to other areas such as the bones, lymph nodes or the brain.

Radiotherapy following lumpectomy or partial mastectomy

Seven research studies from Canada, the US and Europe have shown that giving radiation after a lumpectomy reduces the chance that cancer will re-grow in the breast. Preventing cancer re-growth also improves survival by a few percent.

Even when it appears that the entire tumor has been removed, thin 'tentacles' of cancer cells have been known to extend several centimeters from the main tumor. For this reason, usually the entire breast is treated with radiation.

To avoid unnecessary radiation to the normal structures underneath such as the lung or heart, the radiation is delivered from side to side across the breast (Figure 21). Careful planning of radiation, including the use of a CT scanner, helps prevent side-effects. Women with cancer spread to the axillary lymph nodes may also receive radiotherapy to the lymph node regions above and below the collarbone (see below).

An additional week or so of radiation may be given to the surgery site. This is called a 'boost'. A boost is not required for all patients. A boost reduces the risk of local recurrence and is given if the risk of re-growth in the breast is higher than average. Women younger than age 50 years or who have cancer very close or at the edge of the tissue removed at surgery have a higher risk of breast cancer recurrence and are often given an additional 'boost' dose of radiation.

Partial Breast Radiation: Is it safe and effective?

Follow up of women treated with lumpectomy has shown that if cancer re-grows in the breast, 70% to 80% of the time, it is within a few centimeters (<1 inch) from the original surgery site. Exceptions are women with diffuse ductal carcinoma in situ, women who had more than one cancer in the breast, those whose cancer had spread to the lymph nodes or women whose tumor was of the lobular type (see Chapter 14).

Research is ongoing to determine if it is safe to use radiation only on the affected part rather than the whole breast. Two advantages of partial breast radiation may be that a smaller part of the body is treated (therefore there is less risk of harm from radiation) and that the treatment can often be completed in a single treatment or one week rather than the three to six weeks that are customary with whole breast radiation therapy. Partial breast radiation may be done with standard radiation machines, with brachytherapy or by delivering a single large dose of radiation with a special machine installed in the operating room at the time of lumpectomy.

A concern with partial breast radiation is that there may be a higher risk of cancer re-growth, especially in the parts of the breast that were not treated with radiation. Large scale studies to compare partial and whole breast radiation were started in 2005 and when complete, may radically change the way women with breast cancer are treated.

Radiotherapy after modified radical mastectomy

Modified radical mastectomy (complete removal of the breast) without radiotherapy achieves local control of breast cancer for approximately 75% to 95% of patients with stage I or II breast cancer. However, depending on the extent and type of cancer, the risk of re-growth on the chest wall or in the lymph nodes can be particularly high and radiation may be recommended after mastectomy. Radiation is usually recommended if the cancer was larger than 5 cm, had invaded the adjacent skin or chest wall muscles, or showed extensive spread to the lymph nodes. In these circumstances, the risk of re-growth is usually greater than 30%. Radiotherapy substantially reduces this chance of recurrence.

Until recently it was thought that radiation did not improve life expectancy. However, in the mid-1990s long-term follow-up of research studies comparing radiation to no radiation after mastectomy, demonstrated that radiation added after mastectomy can improve survival for some patients. The benefit, however, is modest: a 5% to 8% increase in survival for women with cancer spread to their lymph nodes who live 10 to 15 or more years after the diagnosis of breast cancer. This benefit must be balanced against an increased risk of side effects (Chapter 26).

There are differing opinions regarding whether all women with cancer in their lymph nodes should have radiation to the chest wall and lymph node regions. Balancing the potential benefits and the risk of increased long-term side effects requires consideration of the characteristics and extent of the cancer in the breast and axilla, the woman's current health, the extent of axillary surgery done and whether there are any signs of arm swelling or other complications after the surgery. The more extensive the cancer and the greater the number of cancer-involved lymph nodes, the more worthwhile it is to have radiation therapy. For patients with one to three lymph nodes containing cancer, additional factors such as the presence of grade 3 disease, cancer found in the lymphatic channels or blood vessels in the breast (see Chapter 12, Pathology) and young age of the patient can identify women at higher risk of cancer re-growth.

One also needs to consider the extent of surgery. If more than 10 to 15 lymph nodes were removed or if the woman already has some arm or hand swelling or a history of heart of lung problems, the chance of serious side effects from the radiation may outweigh any benefits. Women with cancer spread to their lymph nodes should expect to discuss these issues with their radiation oncologist. Whether to use radiation to the regional nodes in addition to chemotherapy, Herceptin® and hormone treatments, is a particularly difficult balance for women with just one to three involved axillary lymph nodes.

Radiotherapy for locally extensive cancer

At the time of diagnosis some women already have a cancer that is considered too extensive to treat with surgery, or for some medical reason, certain women are considered to be unfit for surgery. These women usually receive chemotherapy or hormone therapy depending on their tumor type, age and fitness for withstanding treatment. In addition they usually receive radiation to the breast and the nearby lymph nodes. As a result of these treatments, the cancer may shrink to a size that makes surgery possible.

Radiotherapy for recurrence and relief of symptoms from metastases

Radiotherapy can be especially useful to improve the quality of life of patients who have recurrent cancer or who suffer from symptoms caused by cancer that has spread to other areas of the body (metastases). In these situations, the radiation works by killing cancer cells, thereby shrinking the cancer lumps, and relieving pain and other symptoms. Pain caused by breast cancer metastases in the bones can be relieved in approximately 75% of cases. When there are metastases in the brain, lymph nodes near the breast or some other sites, improvement of symptoms occurs in about 50% of cases.

Radiotherapy is not usually used when the cancer has spread to the lung tissue or the liver because the dose of radiation necessary to kill the cancer cells in these areas is too high for the organs to tolerate. In these situations, hormones, chemotherapy, Herceptin® or a combination of these treatments is used (see Chapter 39).

CHAPTER TWENTY-SIX

Side effects of radiation therapy

What radiotherapy does NOT cause

RADIATION TREATMENTS ARE USUALLY PAINLESS. Some people may experience nausea if a very large area of the body is treated. You will not lose your hair unless the radiation is specifically directed at your head. Except when brachytherapy is used (insertion of radiation sources directly into the breast, see Chapter 24), you are NOT radioactive and you are not a threat to your friends, family or pets. Radiation does not make you dizzy or lightheaded. You should feel well enough to drive yourself back and forth to the clinic for your treatments. Some women even continue full-time employment during radiation treatment.

You may feel tired

The response to radiation is quite variable but most people experience some fatigue. About one woman in three will become noticeably tired. The cause is not known, but the best remedy is to have an afternoon nap, maintain a balanced diet, and cut back on stressful activities. After the radiation treatment is finished, the fatigue decreases gradually over several weeks or months. It is often difficult to tell whether the fatigue is due to the effects of the treatment or the psychological and emotional stress and the life disruption that a new diagnosis of breast cancer brings to every woman.

Emotional effects

Another effect of going to radiation therapy sessions is the daily reminder of the cancer. Many women report that they feel weepy, depressed, angry or frustrated. Discuss your feelings with your radiation therapist and oncologist. You will find that it is a normal, common reaction. Your sense of frustration could be relieved by asserting some control over the process by altering the timing of your appointments to suit you better or simply by expressing concerns and asking questions.

Side effects in the treated breast

The skin

After a partial mastectomy, it is usual for the entire breast, skin and chest wall underneath to be treated with radiation. During several weeks of treatment, the skin gradually becomes pink, red or sun burnt and sometimes eventually peels. Afterwards, the skin may appear tanned. This usually disappears slowly but some women are left with slightly darker skin. Occasionally the skin may blister, usually around the nipple or in the crease beneath the breast. Over time the areola on the treated breast may become pale.

Toward the end of a course of radiation therapy the skin tends to become dry and this causes itchiness. In the past, women were told to keep the skin dry with a dusting of cornstarch. Today it is recognized that the skin feels much better and radiation reactions are actually reduced, if the skin is kept moist. It is recommended that you apply a moisturizing cream two to three times a day during radiation unless the skin breaks down. A hydrocortisone cream can also reduce the sense of burning as the radiation reaction builds up. If the skin cracks or blisters, it is often helpful to apply a commercial antibiotic cream such as Flamazine® (silver sulfadiazine) unless you are allergic to sulfa drugs. If the skin has a severe or painful reaction or breaks down, you should speak to your radiation therapist or nurse.

After the radiation treatment is finished, continued use of a moisturizing cream will reduce the itching and help to lift off any dead or peeling skin, especially around the nipple, which may remain crusty for several months.

Breast firmness

You may notice that the treated breast will be slightly more firm than the untreated one. Radiation can cause the breast to become enlarged, tender, or heavy with fluid during treatment. This may last for six to 18 months afterwards. This is particularly a problem if the breast is swollen, red, infected or heavily bruised after the surgery. It is advised that you continue to wear a bra during treatment and for several months afterwards while the breast is still tender. Don't wear a bra that is constricting or leaves indentations in the breast. The most comfortable bra is often a cotton 'sport bra' without much elastic material and without lace or seams.

'Electric shocks,' prominent blood vessels and scarring

It is normal to experience occasional sharp 'electric shock' sensations in the breast or chest wall. This is NOT a sign of cancer. These fleeting pains are from nerves, damaged during surgery, trying to repair themselves. Red 'spidery' blood vessels may appear 18 to 24 months or more after treatment. This is called telangiectasia. While potentially unsightly, these are NOT a sign of cancer.

Rarely, radiation may cause severe scarring and fibrosis, with discomfort and deformity of the breast. Women who have a lot of swelling, bruising or infection of the breast after surgery are more prone to develop permanent scarring. Also, a small percentage of women (less than 1%) will develop significant scarring for no known reason. In addition, a small percentage of women may have prolonged breast tenderness.

Side effects of treating lymph nodes with radiation

The throat

If the lymph nodes near the collarbone are treated, part of the throat and the top of the lung will be in the path of the radiation beam. You may experience a temporary sore or 'scratchy' throat or the feeling of a 'lump' in the throat. These symptoms are NOT cancer, they are just part of the treatment!

The lungs

Sometimes the lung becomes inflamed a few weeks to several months after the radiation treatment. This reaction is called 'radiation pneumonitis.' If you develop this condition, you will experience a dry, persistent cough, fatigue and, in some cases, fever and chest pain. The pneumonitis usually clears by itself after three to six months, but treatment with steroids may improve symptoms if they are severe.

The heart

Some, but not all, studies of women who have lived 15 or more years after breast cancer treatment, have shown that women treated with radiation for left-sided breast cancer have a small increased chance of having a heart attack. This is because a small portion of the heart may be included in the radiation fields especially when the lymph nodes need to be treated. In these cases radiation may accelerate hardening of the arteries in the heart.

Scarring under the arm

Radiation may increase the amount of scarring caused by surgery in the axilla (armpit). In turn, this may cause scarring in the lymphatic channels and increase the chance of developing arm swelling. It is important to work at regaining full use of your shoulder and, on a permanent basis, to pay careful attention to hand and arm care when the axilla is treated with both surgery and radiation therapy.

Scarring on the chest wall

If radiation is given to the chest wall after mastectomy it can cause some firmness and scarring in the skin and underlying tissues. Approximately 25% of women will have some mild to moderate discomfort in the rib cage even years after radiation, and feel more tenderness if bumped on the treated side. Rarely, radiation may cause a rib to crack or break. If radiation is given after reconstruction with a breast prostheses (Chapter 34), there is more chance of scarring around the prosthesis. This may make the breast mound hard and it can retract up the chest wall toward the collarbone.

Does radiation therapy itself cause cancer?

Low doses of radiation may cause cancer especially in people younger than age 20. However, the high doses used for breast cancer therapy have a low risk of causing cancer. An uncommon form of skin cancer called an angiosarcoma has been reported to develop in the treatment area in somewhat fewer than one in every 1,000 women who survive more than ten years after initially being treated for cancer. This risk needs to be compared to the chance that radiation will prevent the re-growth of the breast cancer— often 100 to 200 or more women per 1,000 receiving radiation will benefit by avoiding re-growth of the breast cancer. There is conflicting evidence about whether radiation therapy for breast cancer increases the risk of other cancers but some studies have shown a very small increased risk of lung or skin cancer in women surviving 10 to 20 years after the treatment of their breast cancer.

SECTION TEN

Chemotherapy

CHAPTER TWENTY-SEVEN

Chemotherapy: What is it?

'CHEMOTHERAPY' MEANS THE USE of any drug or medication to treat disease. For example, antibiotics are a type of chemotherapy. Today, however, the word 'chemotherapy' has come to refer specifically to the cell-killing (cytotoxic) drugs that are used for treating cancer. There are dozens of different chemotherapy (anticancer) drugs. Because they work in different ways, several may be given at once ('combination therapy').

The advantage of chemotherapy is that it travels in the blood stream, reaching cancer cells that may be in distant organs. In contrast, surgery and radiation are local treatments that target one area only.

Chemotherapy is used in three ways in treating breast cancer: 1) as adjuvant treatment to prevent recurrence; 2) as the main or primary treatment for advanced (high-risk) cancers; 3) and to relieve symptoms from cancer that has spread (metastatic cancer).

Chemotherapy as adjuvant treatment

Many patients with breast cancer receive chemotherapy after their surgery if their pathology report (see Chapter 12) indicates that there is a risk of the cancer recurring in other parts of the body. Chemotherapy added to the surgery reduces the chance of recurrence from cancer cells that cannot be detected but are presumed to still be in the body. The concept of adjuvant (preventive) therapy is discussed more completely in Chapter 22.

Chemotherapy as initial treatment for advanced (high-risk) cancer

Chemotherapy is sometimes used before surgery. The delivery of chemotherapy (or hormone therapy) prior to surgery is called 'neoadjuvant' treatment. Neoadjuvant therapy is used if the cancer is too bulky to be removed cleanly at surgery or the surgery would require the removal of too much normal tissue. Locally advanced cancers are either: a) a breast tumor larger than 5.0 cm in diameter and not easily removed by surgery; b) a tumor fixed (tethered firmly) to the chest wall muscles, the rib cage or growing into the skin; or c) a tumor of any size associated with large, suspicious-feeling lymph nodes in the armpit.

Usually, a locally advanced cancer is treated with a combination of chemotherapy and radiation. Once the cancer has become smaller, surgery can be performed to decrease the chance of the cancer recurring in the breast. Inflammatory breast cancer (see Chapter 14) is usually treated in this way as well. Neoadjuvant chemotherapy is also used in cancers that are not locally advanced but are aggressive. Studies have shown that survival is the same if the chemotherapy is given before or after surgery, but surgery may be done earlier if it is given before (neoadjuvant).

Chemotherapy for treating metastatic cancer

If the breast cancer has already spread from the breast, chemotherapy may be used to slow its growth, to decrease symptoms that are caused by the cancer, to improve the patient's quality of life and to prolong the woman's life. A detailed discussion of the treatment of metastatic cancer, including the use of chemotherapy, is included in Chapter 39.

How long does chemotherapy take?

Adjuvant or neoadjuvant chemotherapy is usually prescribed for a three to six-month period. The drugs may be given intravenously (Figure 23) on one day followed by a 14 to 21 day drug-free 'rest period' and then repeated. Some chemotherapy programs use a

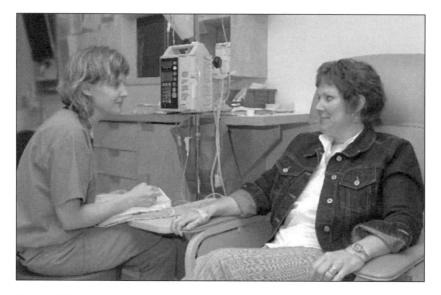

Figure 23: Getting ready for chemotherapy.

combination of oral and intravenous drugs. The alternating treatment and rest periods allow for the maximum cancer-killing effect of the drugs while permitting the body's blood cell counts to return to normal levels during the rest periods (see Chapter 29 on side effects of chemotherapy).

'But I've heard 'horror stories' about chemotherapy!'

Chemotherapy has a bad name due to the severe side effects people used to experience when these drugs were first being developed. Because of these problems, a number of new drugs have been developed to control or eliminate many of these side effects. They are given at the same time as the chemotherapy drugs, improving the patient's well-being while the chemotherapy goes to work on the cancer cells.

Fear also stems from patients not having a clear idea of WHY chemotherapy is being given. If chemotherapy is recommended as a part of your treatment, it is important for you to fully understand the reasons for it and to ask the following questions:

- Why is the oncologist suggesting it?
- What are the goals of the chemotherapy treatment program?

- How long will the treatment take?
- What do I do if I have side effects?
- What are the expected side effects?
- What chemotherapy drugs are being prescribed?
- Who should I call if I have problems?

Once you understand the reasons behind the oncologist's choice of chemotherapy, and you know what to expect, it is easier to accept some side effects knowing that the treatment is the best possible choice for your particular situation.

Mathematical Models to Predict Risk and Benefit

A number of mathematical models have been developed to help health care professionals more accurately assess a woman's risk of recurrence. These can also be helpful in the discussion between the health care professional and the woman as they may provide an easy to understand graph showing an estimate of both the risk of recurrence and the benefit of adjuvant systemic therapy. One frequently used model may be found at www.adjuvantonline.com. The model produces estimates of the chance of recurrence if the patient is treated with surgery alone or treated also with hormonal or chemotherapy. The estimates are based on the best available current data but are just that, estimates only and are very dependent on accurate information being entered about the pathology and extent of the cancer at the time of diagnosis. As such the model should only be used as an aid to and not a replacement for, the consultation.

CHAPTER TWENTY-EIGHT

Who benefits from chemotherapy?

CHEMOTHERAPY MAY BE GIVEN in addition to surgery and radiation when there is a fairly high risk of the cancer recurring. Chemotherapy is not simply given to everyone because there are side effects to the therapy. There must be a winning balance between the possibility of benefit and the risk of side-effects.

The risk of cancer recurrence varies with many factors, some of which we understand and some of which we don't. Table 7 groups patients into broad categories of low, medium, and high risk which clarifies why certain types of therapy are offered to different patients.

Recommendations for adjuvant (post-operative) chemotherapy

Adjuvant chemotherapy is recommended if one or more of the following situations is present:
- axillary lymph nodes contain cancer cells
- the tumor is more than 1 cm in size and high grade (grade 3)
- the tumor is more than 2 cm in size and low or moderate grade (grades 1 and 2)
- tumors with cancer cells that have invaded the lymphatic or vascular channels of the breast are present
- the woman is 35 years old or less even without other risk factors

Table 7 **Basis for recommendations for adjuvant chemotherapy**		
Lowest risk (10% risk of recurrence after 10 years without therapy)	**Moderate risk** (10–20% risk of recurrence after 10 years)	**High risk** (more than 20% risk of recurrence after 10 years)
All of: Tumor less than 1 cm plus no cancer in nodes plus no invasion into lymphatic or blood vessels of the breast	**All of:** Tumor 1–2 cm and grade 1 or 2 plus no cancer in nodes plus no invasion into lymphatic or blood vessels of the breast	**Any one of:** Tumor more than 2 cm, or more than 1 cm and grade 3 and/or nodes contain cancer and/or invasion of lymphatic or blood vessels in the breast
Treatment: No adjuvant chemotherapy; consider hormonal treatment if ER or PR positive*	**Treatment:** Hormone treatment if ER or PR positive* Chemotherapy if ER negative Age less than 35 HER2 overexpression	**Treatment:** Adjuvant chemotherapy, plus hormone therapy if ER or PR positive* Intensive adjuvant chemotherapy, plus hormone therapy if ER or PR positive*
*ER = estrogen receptor, PR = progesterone receptor		

Chemotherapy may be recommended more frequently when tumors are estrogen receptor-negative, as they respond less well to hormonal therapy.

The decision to use chemotherapy depends upon the extent of the cancer, the tumor's estrogen receptors, the other options available for therapy, and the woman's age (older women may not tolerate chemotherapy as well) and the general state of her health. Considering all these factors, women may be offered chemotherapy if their cancer has a moderate or high-risk (see Table 7).

Why is chemotherapy recommended for these women?

Cancer-involved lymph nodes

Cancerous lymph nodes in the armpit indicate a moderate or high risk of cancer recurrence. Surgery alone will cure only a minority of these women because the cancer cells have usually escaped outside the breast before surgery.

However, chemotherapy is not a guarantee. Approximately four women in ten will have a long-term benefit from chemotherapy when it is included with surgery and radiotherapy. However, these numbers are very general and don't tell the whole story: women with few cancer-involved lymph nodes have fewer recurrences than women who have many nodes involved. Also, newer chemotherapy programs may be more effective than the ones used in older studies, so today more women may be cured than in the past.

Since there is no reliable way of knowing exactly which women will be cured by chemotherapy, it is recommended for all premenopausal women with cancerous lymph nodes of the armpit and may also benefit many postmenopausal women.

What about patients whose lymph nodes are free of cancer?

Approximately seven out of ten women with no cancer in their lymph nodes will be cured by surgery and radiation. However, in the other three, breast cancer will recur. When the lymph nodes are negative it becomes important to look at other risk factors to identify women at a high risk of relapse who may benefit from adjuvant chemotherapy. The pathology report contains valuable information about the cancer (see Chapter 12) and its possibility of recurrence, and should be used in making the decision of whether to recommend chemotherapy.

Cancer invading the lymphatics and veins of the breast

If the pathologist sees cancer cells in the lymphatic channels or veins of the breast, there is a higher risk that the cancer has spread beyond the breast. Adjuvant chemotherapy is recommended if the pathology report describes cancer cells in these areas.

A large cancer

The size of the cancer is very important. A 1.0 cm cancer is made up of about one billion cells. The larger the cancer, the higher the risk that some of these cancer cells will have escaped and be growing outside the breast.

Grade of the cancer

Studies have shown that cancers that look aggressive under the microscope (grade 3, see page 90) may recur more frequently.

Women with grade 3 cancers that are greater than 1 cm in size may benefit from chemotherapy.

HER2

Women with tumors that have too much HER2 (overexpression) may have an increased risk of recurrence and may be offered chemotherapy even if there are no other high risk features. Herceptin®, an anti-HER2 antibody is also useful if the woman's tumor overexpresses HER2.

Age

Women younger than 35 years of age often have a more aggressive cancer. Chemotherapy and hormonal therapies may be recommended just because of her young age.

When hormone therapy is less likely to work

In some cases, women with small tumors that are estrogen receptor-negative (poor responders to hormone therapy) and high grade may be judged to be at high enough risk of recurrence to consider adjuvant chemotherapy.

What's best for you

As the understanding of breast cancer improves there will be changes in the recommended treatment. As well, treatment policies may vary somewhat in different centers. Apart from these changes, what is most important is for you to understand why chemotherapy has or hasn't been chosen for your particular case and for you to feel confident that the best possible choice of treatment has been made.

CHAPTER TWENTY-NINE

Side effects of chemotherapy

Why are there side effects?

ALL DRUGS, EVEN ANTIBIOTICS or headache tablets, have potential side effects. What counts is that the beneficial effects of a drug outweigh the problems or discomforts of its side effects. Knowing that a particular drug or combination of drugs can effectively destroy the cancer, you may be more willing to tolerate the side effects, especially if they're temporary.

It is important to be aware of possible side effects before beginning treatment and to discuss them with your doctor. This will make the chemotherapy process less mysterious and frightening and allow you to decide for yourself whether the benefits warrant the side effects.

Although a number of side effects are predictable, others are not. For example, some chemotherapy drugs always cause hair loss while other drugs rarely affect the hair. Different people can also have different reactions to the same drug. In the last few years a number of drugs have become available which have decreased the most feared side effects—nausea and vomiting.

Drug names and drug combinations

An important point to note about drug names is that all drugs have two names: a 'chemical' or 'generic' name, and a brand name.

For example, headache tablets have brand names such as Aspirin® and Tylenol®, but the chemical name for Aspirin® is acetylsalicylic acid and that of Tylenol® is acetaminophen. When you are discussing a particular drug with your doctor, ask him or her to tell you both the chemical name and the brand name (write them down). Since the two names are often referred to interchangeably, being aware of both will avoid confusion.

Different chemotherapy drugs work in different ways. To take maximum advantage of this, the drugs are often given in combinations—attacking on all fronts. Because certain combinations are used frequently, you may see them referred to as abbreviations. Some typical examples are:

- CEF (or FEC): cyclophosphamide, epirubicin and 5-FU
- AC: Adriamycin® and cyclophosphamide
- AC-Taxol®: Adriamycin®, cyclophosphamide and paclitaxel
- CAF (or FAC): cyclophosphamide, Adriamycin® and 5-FU
- TAC or AC-Docetaxel (Taxotere®, Adriamycin®, cyclophosphamide)

All of the above drug names are chemical (generic) names except for the brand names Adriamycin® (its chemical name is doxorubicin), Taxotere® (chemical name is docetaxel) and Taxol® (the chemical name is paclitaxel).

The side effects

Hair loss

Losing your hair is often the most difficult part of chemotherapy. At the doses used, some of the drugs such as doxorubicin, epirubicin, paclitaxel and docetaxel cause baldness in everyone if given at a high enough dose. Other drugs such as cyclophosphamide (Cytoxan®) cause more variable hair loss from thinning or total baldness and others such as 5-FU cause almost no hair loss at all.

Hair loss occurs because the chemotherapy slows down the rapidly dividing cells of the roots of the hair. Thinning usually begins about two weeks after the first dose of chemotherapy. You will notice that you are shedding in the shower, on your brush, and on your pillow. The hair breaks at or near the skin, so the scalp may be tender. The chemotherapy may also cause thinning of the hair on the rest of your body, including your eyebrows, eyelashes, arms, legs and pubic hair. The hair ALWAYS grows back, sometimes even during the chemotherapy, and it is usually already a few inches long by the third month after finishing the drugs.

Hair loss is the most upsetting event for both women and men as it is a public symbol of your cancer. In most situations it cannot be avoided, but fortunately it is temporary. Buy a wig before it happens and take it to your hairdresser to get it styled so you are prepared. If you have long hair, a couple of gradual haircuts could make the change less startling for yourself and your family. Hats, turbans and scarves can be very helpful.

Although there have been attempts to decrease hair loss by scalp hypothermia (cold packs on the scalp) or electrical stimulation of the scalp, these are generally uncomfortable and ineffective. Furthermore, because the cold decreases blood flow to the area, many doctors are concerned that the amount of chemotherapy delivered to that area will be reduced, possibly leaving a potential cancer site untreated.

Infection

White blood cells in the blood stream protect the body from infection. After each injection, many chemotherapy drugs reduce the white blood cell count. If it drops too much, your body's defense mechanisms are low and you have a higher risk of getting an infection.

How can you protect yourself? You don't need to become a hermit but you should take precautions: avoid crowds and contagious diseases such as chickenpox, wash hands frequently, practice good skin care with frequent showers or baths, use a soft toothbrush, use an electric shaver rather than a razor, report painful conditions in the anal area, and be on the alert for any signs of an infection. If you get a fever, sweats, chills, a cough with yellow or green phlegm, burning urine, a sore that will not heal, diarrhea or any other signs of an infection, you should call your doctor immediately so antibiotics can be prescribed. It is rare to require hospitalization, but oral antibiotics may be needed for about five to seven days until your white blood cells recover.

The white cell count usually recovers about 21 days after chemotherapy, which is why many courses of chemotherapy are given in sessions separated by three-week 'holidays'. If your white cell count hasn't recovered enough to make it safe to give another dose of chemotherapy according to the schedule, then treatment will be delayed or the doses will be reduced.

A hormone called 'granulocyte colony stimulating factor' (G-CSF, Neupogen®, Filgrastim®, Pentagastrin®) may be prescribed if you have problems with infection, a very low white blood cell count or if you need frequent doses of chemotherapy. This is a synthetic form of a natural hormone which helps your bone marrow recover and increases your white blood cell count after it has been lowered with chemotherapy. G-CSF is given as an injection under the skin (subcutaneously), similar to an insulin injection, either by the patient or a nurse every day for three to 14 days. Pentagastrin® is a long acting formulation and can be given once every two or three weeks.

Anemia

The number of red blood cells in the blood stream may also be affected by chemotherapy, but it does not usually drop too much.

Anemia may cause you to feel tired, dizzy, short of breath or chilly, so if you notice any of these symptoms you should report them to your doctor. Although you should eat well, anemia caused by chemotherapy is not usually helped by taking iron or B vitamins since the low red cell count is not caused by nutritional deficiencies but by a decreased production of red cells. If your anemia becomes severe enough to cause symptoms, (often when the hemoglobin falls to less than 100g/L) your doctor may recommend a blood transfusion or an injection of a hormone called 'erythropoeitin' (Epo®, Epogen®) which may help stimulate your bone marrow to make more red blood cells.

Abnormal bleeding or bruising

Platelets help to clot the blood. Chemotherapy may cause a temporary decrease of the platelet count. If this is severe enough, you may bleed easily. It is rare for low platelet counts to be a significant problem, but if you notice any abnormal bleeding or bruising you should report it to your doctor. ASA (Aspirin®) or Ibuprofen (Advil®) drugs can slow down platelet function and should be taken only after checking with your doctor. However, acetaminophen (Tylenol®) does not affect the platelets and is generally all right to take in moderation.

Nausea and vomiting

Most of the chemotherapeutic drugs can cause nausea and vomiting, although some people are affected more than others. 'Antiemetic' drugs, which prevent nausea and vomiting, are usually given before the chemotherapy and every few hours afterwards for the first 24 to 48 hours. The nausea may start six to eight hours after the chemotherapy injection, or even the next day, and is usually not a prolonged problem. Eat something before the chemotherapy and regularly thereafter because it is often better not to have an empty stomach.

The nausea may feel like morning sickness, so it is sometimes helpful to take an antiemetic, have something to eat (for instance some dry crackers) and stay in bed for an hour to prevent vomiting. Avoid odors that cause more nausea. If the drugs you are given are not effective, tell your doctor so that different or additional antiemetics can be tried.

The drugs used to prevent nausea and vomiting include ondansetron (Zofran®), prochlorperazine (Stemetil®), dimenhydrinate (Gravol®), metoclopramide (Maxeran®, Nabilone®), and dexamethasone (Decadron®). Diphenhydramine (Benadryl®) and lorazepam (Ativan®) may also be helpful. Note that these drugs may also have side effects. For example, ondansetron (Zofran®) may cause headaches and constipation and prochlorperazine (Stemetil®) may cause restlessness that could require yet another drug, diphenhydramine (Benadryl®), for relief. The drugs may be given as pills, intravenous or intramuscular medications or rectal suppositories. The suppositories may be the easiest to take if you are vomiting or nauseated.

Some people also complain about stomach pain, an acidy feeling, heartburn, and a change in the taste in their mouth. These symptoms may be eased by food or antacids, but if the symptoms are severe, particularly the pain, you should notify your doctor.

Diarrhea and constipation

The anti-cancer drugs often cause some change in your bowel habits so don't be alarmed by minor disruptions. If you have severe diarrhea for more than 24 hours, or cramps, you should call your doctor because an anti-diarrheal drug may stop the problem. As well, you should be assessed to make sure this was actually related to the chemotherapy and not something totally unrelated. A stool culture may be necessary to ensure that you do not have an infection. If you have diarrhea, try to drink lots of clear liquids to replace the fluid that you have lost and to rest your bowels. Avoid foods such as cabbage, beans, brans and spicy foods that cause loose bowels, gas and cramps. Milk products may also contribute to diarrhea.

Some chemotherapy drugs may cause constipation. Often this can be avoided by drinking plenty of fluids, keeping active and possibly taking a mild stool softener. If you have a severe problem, notify your doctor.

Sore mouth (mucositis)

Many of the chemotherapy drugs cause soreness or dryness of the mouth and throat that can appear about five days after treatment begins. If this is a problem, avoid foods that irritate your mouth such as acidic, spicy or rough foods. Rinse your mouth often with baking soda and water. If your mouth gets so sore that you cannot eat, notify your doctor, as there are mouthwashes and painkillers that may ease your discomfort. People who tend to get cold sores (herpes) in addition to other mouth sores can be helped by an antiviral medication. If a white, cakey covering develops in your mouth you may have a yeast infection (candida) which can cause mouth soreness and difficulty eating and swallowing. A special mouthwash or pill may help.

Menstrual periods and sexuality

Chemotherapy may disrupt your menstrual periods, causing them to be irregular, to stop temporarily during chemotherapy and then return, or to stop permanently. This is not predictable, but it is more likely to happen in women closer to menopause than in younger women or if you are taking six months of chemotherapy rather than three months (see Menopause, below). If you are having menstrual changes, discuss them with your oncologist.

Chemotherapy drugs generally do not affect the ability to have sex, although you may notice changes. The mucosal lining of the vagina may feel dry or sore. A vaginal lubricant such as Replens® is helpful. As well, you might be at risk of getting a yeast (candida) infection which may irritate the area and may require treatment with antifungal creams. Certain sexual positions could cause discomfort to your arm or chest area after surgery. Your libido, or sexual desire, may be affected by the stress of the illness, fatigue, your anxiety and the changes in your body which may affect your hormones, self-confidence and your body image. These are natural and normal responses that may be temporary. If you have continued difficulties with your sexual interest or activity, you and possibly your partner may want to discuss strategies to rekindle your sexuality with a professional counselor.

Menopause

Menopause is simply when menstrual periods stop completely, and is usually defined as one year without periods. We now know that the hormonal changes that occur with menopause normally develop over a decade or so. At menopause the ovaries stop releasing eggs and make less estrogen. This decrease in the level of estrogen causes changes in the body in a wide variety of organs and tissues. In some women these changes are subtle and do not cause any problems. In other women they are troublesome and cause upsetting and frustrating symptoms.

Chemotherapy can bring on an early and abrupt menopause in some women due to the effect of the drugs on the ovaries. This is more common in women over the age of 40 and may depend on which drugs are used and the total doses prescribed. In some women the periods stop temporarily; in others they stop permanently. Even with blood tests and symptoms, it is sometimes difficult to know how complete the menopause is for six months to one year. The symptoms of menopause are often a distressing part of the cancer treatment.

Menopause is a natural occurrence. It can be associated with the following symptoms and changes:
- dry skin
- dryness of the vagina and perineum
- hot flashes
- weight gain
- mood changes
- increased risk of osteoporosis (thin bones, decrease in the calcium content of the bones. Is called osteopenia when it is mild and osteoporosis when more severe. May be associated with an increased risk of bone fractures)

- increased risk of heart disease
- memory changes
- changes in libido (interest in sex).

Menopause is not the same for all women. It is important to have a discussion with your doctor about the symptoms you are having in context with your family history. If women in your family have a significant history of developing heart disease or osteoporosis at a young age, there may be specific precautions that you should start early. As well, your doctor may want to assess your bones with a bone density test. This test is like a bone scan but shows whether there is evidence of osteopenia or osteoporosis.

To avoid some of the problems associated with menopause:

- Stop smoking. It can cause heart disease, osteoporosis, lung disease and cancer.
- Do some exercise. Weight-bearing exercise can protect against osteoporosis; cardiopulmonary exercise is important for your heart and weight.
- Check your diet. Ensure that you have 1500 to 2000 mg of calcium in your diet or as supplements, 300 IU of vitamin D, and a low-fat, low-cholesterol diet.
- For vaginal dryness: a water-soluble lubricating jelly (e.g. Replens®) can help make intercourse less painful. Occasionally, estrogen creams may be used sparingly. Estring® is an intravaginal low-dose estrogen.
- If you have hot flashes, try to reduce your stress, and limit your intake of caffeine, alcohol, chocolate, and cola, as they can worsen hot flashes. Hot flashes may also be decreased with vitamin E, evening primrose oil, Remifemin® (black cohosh) or other herbal remedies. Prescription drugs that may help include Effexor®, Dixarit®, Bellagral®, low-dose Megace®. The use of estrogens and progesterones (Megace® is a type of progesterone) for women with a history of breast cancer remains controversial but these medications are being studied to assess their safety.
- Osteoporosis may be treated with medications such as biphosphonates (etidronate, clodrinate, Fosamax®), which decrease the bone changes, and occasionally with progesterones and estrogens. New agents such as raloxifene may be effective but should not be used without consultation with an oncologist.

Preliminary studies suggest it may protect against osteoporosis, heart disease, and possibly breast cancer.

- For changes in libido: It may just take time to get used to your body's changes. Occasionally, testosterone is recommended, as it may help encourage your sexual interest. Because testosterone can be converted into estrogen in your body, its use after a diagnosis of breast cancer, especially if ER positive, is controversial.

Discuss your symptoms and concerns with your doctor.

It is important to remember that there is not one solution for all women. Menopausal changes and concerns are very variable.

Prevent pregnancy during chemotherapy, but not with 'the pill'

Taking chemotherapy does not necessarily prevent pregnancy. Furthermore, IT IS IMPORTANT NOT TO GET PREGNANT WHILE ON CHEMOTHERAPY because these drugs, especially during the first three months of pregnancy, may cause damage and deformity of the fetus. While on chemotherapy, it is important to continue to use birth control measures; these should be discussed with your doctor. As your periods could be irregular, it may be difficult to predict the time of ovulation, so a combination of a barrier method (a condom or diaphragm) plus a spermicidal foam or gel is safest. Oral contraceptives are generally NOT recommended if you have breast cancer because estrogens are believed to stimulate some cancers.

Many women ask about having a baby after they have finished chemotherapy. If you continue to have periods and ovulate you may be able to get pregnant, but you should wait until you are fully recovered from the treatment and until you and your oncologist have discussed the risk of the cancer coming back. Pregnancy itself will not cause the cancer to come back, but the unpredictable nature of breast cancer and its potential for recurrence needs to be considered prior to a pregnancy.

If you are pregnant when you are diagnosed with breast cancer, chemotherapy may be given if you are in your second or third trimester and if it is important to begin treatment right away.

General symptoms

All of the drugs may cause skin changes such as dryness, spots, increased sun sensitivity, or rashes. If you're going out in the sun, wear protective clothing, including a sun hat. Many women complain about dry, gritty eyes which can be eased by eye drops or artificial tears. Other women complain of a flu-like feeling or of feeling cold for one to three days after the chemotherapy starts.

If the drug contains a dye (for example Adriamycin®, which is red) your urine may change color the day after you start chemotherapy as you excrete the drug. You do not need to take special precautions in the bathroom, as the chemotherapy drugs are not dangerous to anyone else. You should drink plenty of fluids to ensure a good urine flow and to prevent bladder irritation.

Some women develop joint or muscle aches and pains. These often begin after the chemotherapy is finished and can last several months. Fortunately, they are usually temporary and can be relieved with exercise or anti-inflammatory medications.

Certain drugs may cause tingling in the fingers and toes, and some people report a loss of muscle strength and a change in their sense of balance. This also should be temporary. If it is not, or if it interferes with your activities, report it to your doctor.

Some women complain of 'chemo brain', a loss in their short-term memory. This is often temporary. Studies have confirmed that some impairment of memory loss may occur during or shortly after treatment. It is difficult to know if the memory loss is due to the chemotherapy, the stress of the illness or all the anti-nausea and other medications that are taken. It is also not known if there are any long-term effects (more than two years) or how many women are significantly affected.

If you experience any new problem, report it to your doctor. It may or may not be related to the chemotherapy. If you have finished your treatments and are on follow-up, you should probably report it to your family doctor, since your complaints may be unrelated to the therapy.

Other considerations while taking chemotherapy

While you are on chemotherapy, you can eat whatever you like. However, if you are taking some other medication for another condition, your doctor should verify that it can be continued. Although some physicians and nutritionists recommend total abstinence from alcohol, an occasional glass of wine or beer is usually alright, but check with your doctor.

Fatigue levels vary. Some women are able to continue their normal activities and continue working throughout chemotherapy. Others find chemotherapy so physically or emotionally draining they need to take a leave from work. Although it is recommended that you remain as active as you can while on chemotherapy, you will need some extra rest. Since it's hard to predict how much rest you will need, it may be worthwhile to sit down with your family or your employer and warn them that there will be low-energy days.

Physical activity is important. If you exercise regularly you might want to continue, but tone down your routine to avoid straining yourself. Walks could replace your daily jogs.

Hormone therapy

CHAPTER THIRTY

Hormone therapy:
What is it and who benefits from it?

What are the female hormones?

THE FEMALE HORMONES ESTROGEN and progesterone control many of the female and sex related processes of the body, such as the growth of female genitals and breasts, development of the female body shape and regulation of the menstrual cycle.

What is the relationship between hormones and breast cancer?

Estrogen not only stimulates the growth of the breasts but is also appears to encourage the growth of some, but not all, breast tumors. Progesterone can also simulate the growth of breast tumors.

Do hormone treatments work for all breast cancers?

Hormone treatment is only effective in tumors that have hormone receptors (see Chapter 14). Hormone receptors can be either estrogen receptors (ER) or progesterone receptors (PR) and are found on approximately 70% to 75% of breast cancers. They are measured on the tumor by the pathologist and predict if the tumor will respond to hormone treatment. Most laboratories use an immunoperoxidase method (IHC) and report the amount of

163

receptor in a particular cancer as 0, 1+, 2+, or 3+, where 0 is negative for receptors and 3+ is a high receptor content. In general the higher the estrogen receptor level in the tumor, the more responsive the tumor will be to hormone treatments.

ER or PR: Are they both important?

Estrogen receptors are more frequent and appear to be the more important receptor. Progesterone receptors appear to generally affect how well the estrogen receptor functions. Tumors may have both receptors positive (ER+PR+), just estrogen receptors positive (ER+PR-) or both negative (ER-PR-). With current pathology methods it is very rare to find tumors that are ER-PR+.

What is hormone therapy?

Hormone therapy for breast cancer (sometimes called 'anti-estrogen' therapy) is a form of whole body (systemic) treatment that is used as adjuvant treatment or for cancer recurrence. The term 'hormone therapy' refers to a number of different treatments designed to affect the level of female hormones in the body. These include the use of drugs for both pre-menopausal and post-menopausal women or the removal or destruction of the ovaries in pre-menopausal women by either surgery, medications or radiation.

Changing the hormone levels affects the cancer cells and slows their growth. A number of different drugs can do this effectively. The particular drug chosen depends on whether the woman is pre-menopausal or post-menopausal and the stage of her disease since not all drugs have been proven to be effective for all stages. Hormone therapy is used for prevention, in situ disease, the adjuvant therapy of invasive disease and in recurrent breast cancer. Hormone therapy has been shown to decrease the chance of the cancer coming back both in the affected breast and in the rest of body, and also has been shown to decrease the risk of a new cancer developing in the opposite breast.

A woman with breast cancer is defined as pre-menopausal or post-menopausal based on her menstrual status at the time of treatment. This chapter will focus on general hormone therapy recommendations after surgery. Chapter 31 will discuss side effects. Appendix 2 lists the various hormone therapies.

Hormone therapy in pre-menopausal women

Before menopause, estrogen is made primarily by the ovaries. The pituitary gland, which is in the brain, releases hormones (LH and FSH) that control ovulation, the menstrual cycle and the production of estrogen in the ovaries. Pituitary gland hormones are released based on the level of estrogen in the blood. When the estrogen level goes down FSH is released to stimulate the ovaries. Pituitary hormones are also released at different times during the menstrual cycle. Regular menstrual cycles are a sign of normal ovarian function but do not tell the whole story. Many women's periods get irregular or stop with chemotherapy. But, sometimes ovarian function returns and the ovaries are still able to produce estrogen.

The goal of hormone therapy in breast cancer is to either stop the production of estrogen from the ovaries or stop the effect of the estrogen on the breast cancer cells.

Tamoxifen

Tamoxifen (Novaldex®, Tamofen®, etc.) is effective in stopping the effect of estrogen on the breast cancer cells. Tamoxifen has been shown to be effective in the adjuvant therapy of both in situ and invasive cancers which have hormone receptors. The decision to use tamoxifen in adjuvant therapy is based on the risk of the cancer recurring taking into account the size of the tumor, the involvement of axillary nodes, the grade, the finding of lymphatic or vascular invasion and the hormone receptor status. Since it has been suggested that tamoxifen may be less effective in tumors that overexpress HER2, the HER2 status may be considered as well .

Ovarian suppression

Since the ovaries are producing estrogen in pre-menopausal women, suppressing the ovaries will decrease the estrogen levels. This has been shown to be an effective treatment. Various treatments may put a woman into menopause either permanently or temporarily (side effects discussed in Chapter 31).

Oophorectomy

Oophorectomy is surgical removal of the ovaries which can be done with minimal surgery (laparoscopically) or with a full surgical procedure with or without the removal of the uterus. Removing the uterus does not affect the estrogen levels.

Radiation

Radiation ablation refers to using radiation (usually daily for five days) to permanently damage the ovaries so they stop producing estrogens. It generally takes about three months after radiation to the ovaries will decrease the levels of estrogen to a post-menopausal level.

Pituitary suppression

Drugs called 'LHRH-agonists' interfere with the normal pathway of the pituitary hormones, LH and FSH. By blocking the release of LH and FSH, the ovaries temporarily stop producing estrogen. When the drugs are stopped, the ovaries generally start working normally again. LHRH-agonists are given as an intramuscular injection every month to three months for two to five years when used as adjuvant treatment. These drugs include goserelin (Zoladex®) or buserelin (Suprefact®) and less commonly triptorelin (Trelstar®) and leuprolide (Lupron®). The LHRH-agonists are given on their own or with an oral hormone treatment.

Hormone therapy in post-menopausal women

A woman is defined as post-menopausal when she has not had periods for a year. Women who have had their uterus removed (hysterectomy) but still have their ovaries, are not postmenopausal until their ovaries stop producing estrogen. Menopause may be suspected if the woman has menopausal symptoms such as hot flushes and can be confirmed by blood test for hormone levels. The average age of menopause in North America is 52 years. Since some women experience symptoms of hot flushes, vaginal dryness, mood changes, an increased risk of osteoporosis and skin changes, menopause is often discussed as if it were a disease when in fact, it is simply a normal physiological event.

After menopause a woman still makes estrogen but the levels of estrogen are significantly lower than before menopause. Estrogen is made by the body by a complicated process which involves the adrenal glands, their production of cholesterol, and its eventual change into estrogen. The last enzyme involved in this long process of converting cholesterol to estrogen is called aromatase. The aromatase enzyme is found in a large number of tissues in the body including fat, muscle, liver, breast and breast cancer cells.

In post-menopausal women, hormone sensitive breast cancers can be treated either by blocking the estrogen receptor on the cell (tamoxifen) or by interfering with the aromatase enzyme to stop estrogen production with a group of drugs known as aromatase inhibitors: anastrozole (Arimidex®), letrozole (Femara®) and exemestane (Aromasin®).

Tamoxifen (see above)

As well as decreasing the risk of cancer recurrence, tamoxifen may have other beneficial effects for post-menopausal women. It reduces cholesterol and lipids in the blood which may be good for the heart. Some studies have also shown that women who took tamoxifen had less calcium loss from their bones, fewer fractures and less osteoporosis.

Aromatase inhibitors

The aromatase inhibitors act by blocking the enzyme aromatase and are only effective in women who are truly post-menopausal and not making estrogen in their ovaries. These drugs were initially studied in recurrent disease where they were found to be effective. More recent studies have shown that they are beneficial in early breast cancer as well.

Anastrozole (Arimidex®), letrozole (Femara®) and exemestane (Aromasin®) have all been shown to be effective in early breast cancer by decreasing the chance of the cancer regrowing in the affected breast or elsewhere in the body and by decreasing the chance of a new cancer growing in the other breast. Various studies have been conducted using these drugs instead of tamoxifen, after two to three years of tamoxifen for another two to three years to make up a total of five years and in the case of letrozole, after completing five years of tamoxifen. Ongoing research studies will add to and refine our knowledge of how to best use the aromatase inhibitors. However, if a woman is post-menopausal and has a hormone receptor positive tumor, these drugs should be discussed as an option for adjuvant treatment.

Two studies have reported that longer hormone adjuvant therapy may be helpful. The first and largest study was the MA17 study that added letrozole after five years of tamoxifen. The MA17 showed that women had fewer recurrences by taking the aromatase inhibitor after completing five years of tamoxifen. In a second study, women completing five years of tamoxifen should discuss the use of letrozole with their doctors and decide whether to take it based on the risk of the initial tumor and other health problems. Note that taking tamoxifen for more than five years has been shown to be potentially harmful and is not recommended. Raloxifene (Evista®) is a drug used for osteoporosis which has a chemical structure that is very similar to tamoxifen. There are concerns that it may also affect breast cancer recurrence if taken for more than five years.

Table 8 **Recommendations for the use of adjuvant therapy for hormone sensitive breast cancers**

Lowest risk of recurrence	Moderate risk of recurrence	High risk of recurrence	Extreme risk of recurrence
All of	**All of**	**Any one of**	**Any one of**
Tumor less than 1 cm **Plus** No cancer in lymph nodes **Plus** No invasion into lymph channels or blood vessels of the breast or into lymph nodes **Plus** HER2 normal	Tumor 1–2 cm **Plus** No cancer in lymph nodes **Plus** No invasion into lymph channels or blood vessels of the breast or into lymph nodes and Grade 1–2 histology **Plus** HER2 normal	Tumor more than 2 cm **Or** 1–3 lymph nodes with cancer **Or** Cancer seen in lymph channels or blood vessels of the breast or Grade 1–2 histology +/– HER2 overexpression	Tumor more than 5 cm with cancer in lymph nodes **Or** >3 lymph nodes with cancer **Or** Skin invasion Chest wall invasion Inflammatory cancer +/– HER2 overexpression
Recommendations for Postmenopausal women			
Adjuvant hormone therapy may be nil **Or** Letrozole x 3–5yr Tamoxifen x 5yr **Or** Anastrozole x 5yr **Or** Tam x 2–3yr followed by Exemstane x 2–3yr	Adjuvant hormone therapy with Tamoxifen x 5yr with consideration **Or** Anastrozole x 5yr **Or** Tam x 2–3yr followed by Exemstane x 2–3yr	Adjuvant chemo + Adjuvant hormone therapy with Anastrozole x 5yr **Or** Tam x 2–3yr followed by Exemstane x 2–3yr **Or** Tam x 5yr followed by Letrozole x 3–5yr	Adjuvant chemo + Adjuvant hormone therapy with Anastrozole x 5yr **Or** Tamoxifen x 2–3yr followed by Exemstane x 2–3yr **Or** Tam x 5yr followed by Letrozole x 3–5yr
Recommendations for Pre-menopausal women			
Adjuvant tamoxifen **Or** nil	Adjuvant tamoxifen **Or** LHRH agonist + Tam or AI	Adjuvant chemo + Tamoxifen x 5yr **Or** if postmenopausal Tam x 2–3yr followed by Exemstane x 2–3yr **Or** LHRH agonist x 2–3yr + Tamoxifen Or + Anastrozole	Adjuvant chemo + Tamoxifen x 5yr **Or** after therapy Tam x 2–3yr followed by Exemstane x 2–3yr **Or** LHRH agonist x 2–3yr + Tamoxifen Or + Anastrozole

AI = Aromatase inhibitor (anastrozole, letrozole, exemestane)
Tam = tamoxifen

CHAPTER THIRTY-ONE

Side effects of hormone therapy

Do hormone therapies have side effects?

AS WITH ALL DRUG TREATMENTS, there are potential side effects associated with hormone treatments. These must be carefully discussed and considered before starting treatments. The side effects may depend on the dose and the length of treatment but often vary significantly between individuals. Some women have no side effects while others suffer. This can usually not be predicted. Any treatment must be a balance of benefit and toxicity. If you do have side effects, notify the doctor who prescribed the treatment.

Menopausal Symptoms

Any drug that either causes menopause to occur (LHRH agonists) or drugs that lower estrogen (aromatase inhibitors) can cause the symptoms associated with low body levels of estrogen. Not all women experience symptoms with menopause. Sometimes symptoms are more severe if there is a sudden decrease in the estrogen level, as happens when a woman has her ovaries removed, stops estrogen replacement therapy, or goes into menopause with chemotherapy.

Hot flushes

Hot flushes may be minor or may be severe. They are often temporary and most women report they get better with time. Avoiding triggers such a caffeine (found in coffee, tea, chocolate or colas), alcohol and stress may be beneficial. Although studies have not shown a consistent effect from vitamin E, some women are helped. Plant estrogens such as black cohosh may be helpful, but it is not clear if they (or soy) have sufficient estrogen effects to act on breast cancer cells. Prescription medications such as low doses of antidepressants such as Effexor or Paxil have been shown to reduce the number and severity of hot flashes as has the drug Dixarit (clonidine). Studies of gabapentin also suggest a benefit.

Vaginal dryness and irritation

Vaginal dryness and irritation can make sexual intercourse painful and difficult. Lubricating jellies such as Replens, Muko, Astroglide or Slippery Stuff may be helpful. This jelly can be applied to the vaginal opening and the head of the penis to make intercourse easier. If the symptoms are severe, it is sometimes helpful to use a small amount of estrogen. This may be in the form of an estrogen cream that should be applied sparingly to the opening of the vagina as needed. Estring is an intravaginal ring which slowly releases a low dose of estrogen into the vagina and may decrease dryness and irritation. Although some of the estrogen may be released from either the cream or the ring into the blood stream, it is likely a small amount that has a small risk. Quality of life issues may be more important to a woman and should be discussed.

Osteoporosis and increased risk of fractures

Without estrogen there is a loss of calcium from the bones and the risk of bone fractures and osteoporosis increases. Women who have a family history of osteoporosis, who smoke, drink excessive coffee and alcohol, or who have been on medications such as steroids for a long time have an increased risk of osteoporosis. It is recommended that all pre-menopausal women take in 1000 mg of calcium and 400 IU of Vitamin D per day and that post-menopausal women take in 1500 mg of calcium and 800 IU of Vitamin D per day. Chapter 35 lists foods which contain calcium. Regular weight bearing exercise is also important to bone health.

For women taking an aromatase inhibitor, a baseline bone density should be done and repeated every 18 to 24 months. If there is significant bone loss, these drugs may not be appropriate and treatment with a medication to improve bone density (possibly a bisphosphanate) may be indicated.

Weight gain

Many women gain a few kilograms at the time of menopause. This may also occur if one is taking hormonal therapy for breast cancer.

Tamoxifen

Tamoxifen is an estrogen as well as an anti-estrogen. This means that it acts like an estrogen on some normal tissues but blocks estrogen receptors at the cancer cells. Many women have no side effects with tamoxifen while others report the side effects listed below.

- Hot flashes
- Vaginal discharge: this may be clear or whitish. If it is bloody, you should call your doctor. If it is itchy or has an odor, see your doctor.
- Phlebitis and/or thrombosis: this is an inflamed vein that contains a blood clot. It occurs in about 1% of women taking tamoxifen for five years. If the clot dislodges and travels to other parts of the body, particularly the lung, it can be dangerous. Clots are more common in women who have had a previous clot, who smoke, who are inactive, who are getting chemotherapy at the same time, and who have a family history of clots. If you have a swollen or painful leg or calf muscle, see your doctor. If a diagnosis of a blood clot is made, you may need to be on medications to dissolve the clot and tamoxifen probably should be stopped.
- Continuation of menses: This is common with pre-menopausal women. As ovulation can continue, birth control precautions should be maintained as tamoxifen could be harmful to a fetus.
- Endometrial (uterus) cancer: At the recommended dose of tamoxifen of 20 mg given for five years, approximately two women per 1000 will develop an endometrial cancer each year. This is two to three times higher than the risk for women

172

not taking tamoxifen. However, for women with an invasive breast cancer more than 1 cm in diameter, the chance of developing endometrial cancer while taking tamoxifen is much less than the benefit of avoiding a breast cancer recurrence. If you have any unexplained vaginal bleeding while taking tamoxifen, you should see your doctor.

Very rare side effects include:
- Nausea /vomiting / loss of appetite: usually temporary
- Muscles and joint aches and pains: may be related to menopause.
- Rash / Skin dryness and hair loss
- Headache, depression, dizziness
- Facial hair
- Fatigue and malaise
- Retinal changes: vision changes have been rarely reported. If you notice a change in your vision, you should get your eyes checked by an eye doctor.
- High calcium: occurs rarely when a woman has bone metastases
- Flare up of pain: If there are metastases, these may initially get more painful.

Other anti-estrogens

Faslodex (fulvesant)—This is a new anti-estrogen that is used in recurrent breast cancer. It is given as an intramuscular injection every 28 days. It has only been studied in post-menopausal women. Side effects include:
- Nausea and vomiting
- Constipation, diarrhea, and abdominal pain
- Headache
- Back pain
- Hot flashes
- Pain and swelling where the needle was injected

Raloxifene is a drug that is very similar to tamoxifen. There are ongoing studies to see if it is a good drug for breast cancer prevention but the results of the studies are not yet known. It is not presently used in the treatment of breast cancer.

Aromastase Inhibitors

These drugs are only effective in post-menopausal women as they block an enzyme called aromatase that is the last step in the production of estrogen in post-menopausal women. There are three aromatase inhibitors that are all used in both adjuvant therapy of invasive breast cancer and in recurrent disease. These drugs are anastrozole (Arimidex®), letrozole (Femara®) and exemestane (Aromasin®). They are very similar in activity and in side effects, and at this time it is not clear if there is one drug that will be shown to be more effective than another.

As these drugs decrease estrogen levels, the most common side effects are those associated with menopause. These include hot flushes, vaginal dryness and an increased risk of osteoporosis. This last side effect is the most serious and should be part of the discussion about the risks and benefits of taking treatment, particularly in women with very low risk breast cancers.

Side effects include:
- Muscle and joint aches and pains: these may be mild or more severe and often occur after a woman has been taking an aromatase inhibitor for a while. If they are troublesome, an anti-inflammatory pill such as ibuprofen may be helpful. If they are severe, discuss it with your doctor.
- Increase in lipid and triglyceride levels are seen. These may be of no concern but if you have other risk factors for heart disease such as high blood pressure, a family history or if you are overweight, you should discuss this with your doctor and possibly take a lipid lowering drug.
- Loss of sexual libido: this could be due to a number of causes, including the psychological stresses associated with cancer, but it may be worse while taking these drugs.

Less common side effects include:
- Nausea: this usually is temporary
- Headaches
- Swelling of hands, feet or lower legs if your body retains fluid
- Fatigue and tiredness
- Thinning of the hair is not common but can occur and is usually only mild. If it does occur, it will grow back when you stop taking the drug.

- Skin rash
- Depression
- Weight gain
- Vaginal bleeding or discharge
- Diarrhea
- Trouble sleeping

Inhibitors of the pituitary hormones (LHRH agonists)

These drugs are sometimes used in pre-menopausal women to put the woman into a temporary menopause by stopping the production of estrogen in the ovaries. This is done by blocking release of the hormones from the pituitary gland that controls the ovaries. Studies on a number of these drugs have shown that they are very similar in both their effectiveness and their side effects. Sometimes a combination of an LHRH agonist and tamoxifen is given in addition to chemotherapy or instead of chemotherapy. There are ongoing studies trying to determine the best way to use these drugs and which pre-menopausal women benefit. These studies are also looking at the combination of an LHRH agonist and an aromatase inhibitor in pre-menopausal women.

LHRH agonists include goserelin (Zoladex®), buserelin (Suprefact®), triptorelin (Trelstar®), and leuprolide (Lupron®). These drugs are all given by a subcutaneous injection and are given on a monthly schedule. Some of the drugs have a long acting formulation (a depot) and can be given once every three months.

Side effects include the menopausal symptoms described above. However studies have suggested that if there is bone loss, it is not permanent and after the LHRH agonist is stopped and ovarian function returns, the calcium content of the bones (the bone density) can return to normal.

Other side effects are rare but may include:
- Pain, tenderness or redness where the needle was placed
- Increased bone pain during the first one to two weeks
- Nausea
- Breast swelling and/or soreness
- A decrease in sex drive
- Unexpected vaginal bleeding
- Appetite or bowel changes
- Tiredness, headache, depression, dizziness, irritability

- Difficulty in sleeping
- Numbness or tingling of feet and hands
- Swelling of hands, feet, or lower legs if you retain fluid
- Itchy skin rash
- Bone or joint pain
- Changes in eyesight

Other hormonal agents

There are a number of other hormone drugs that are occasionally used in recurrent breast cancer. These include:

Progestins

Megesterol acetate (Megace) is now used relatively infrequently. It is not clear how this drug works, even though progestins have been used in the treatment of breast cancer for many years. Megace is usually well tolerated but there are some side effects and these may include:
- Significant weight gain: in 20% to 30% of women.
- Vaginal bleeding
- High blood pressure, headaches and depression
- Fluid retention, shortness of breath, increased respiratory rate
- High blood sugar levels
- Nausea and vomiting

Androgens

Androgens are male hormones that can be used to treat recurrent breast cancer. The side effects often depend on the dose, how long the treatment is continued and the individual. Side effects include:
- Masculinizing effects such as scalp hair loss, growth of facial and body hair, lowering of the voice, increase in size of the clitoris.
- Weight gain
- Nausea and decreased appetite.

PART THREE | **Beyond the initial phase of treatment**

Coping with cancer

CHAPTER THIRTY-TWO

Living with a diagnosis of breast cancer: Tips for you, your family and your friends

EVERY PERSON WITH CANCER and every family member is unique, but the road each must travel is well worn by the millions of others who have come before. It is a journey marked by hope and despair, courage and fear, humor, anger and uncertainty.

Is there a 'right way' to feel after receiving a cancer diagnosis?

Many women are concerned that the thoughts and feelings they experience following a diagnosis of cancer are somehow abnormal or crazy and that there must be a 'right way' to feel. This couldn't be further from the truth. There is no one way to feel. Reactions to the diagnosis can span the full range of human emotion: anger, anxiety, uncertainty, hopelessness, helplessness, depression, a feeling of isolation, vulnerability, relief that there really is something wrong, and even guilt that one has somehow contributed to the development of her own disease or delayed in bringing it to a doctor's attention.

It is important to realize that the initial reaction to the diagnosis will be followed by other feelings. Just as we go through a series of 'stages' in accepting the loss of a loved one, we pass through a number of emotional levels on our way to acknowledging the diagnosis of cancer. First, there is often disbelief in the diagnosis, denial that it is true, and anger at being 'singled out.' Finally, there is usually an acknowledgement that 'Yes, I do have cancer.'

Denial is often a prominent response early in the cancer experience. It is a defense against fear and helps to maintain emotional equilibrium. It is not uncommon to hear people comment, 'I think she's in denial,' as if there may be something unusual and potentially dangerous about this reaction. In fact, some degree of denial is normal and is probably necessary to protect oneself and to maintain the hope needed to participate in daily life. However, it is important to recognize that denial is healthy only as long as it does not interfere with seeking medical care or participating in appropriate treatment.

Expressions of very strong emotion are to be expected and they may range from anger and bitterness to frank hostility which may be directed at anyone and anything.

Fortunately, most people will emerge from the storm of emotions to reach a point of equilibrium and acknowledgement. It is common to move back and forth from one 'stage' to another. Many think about having cancer in the past tense which helps to keep the cancer from dominating a woman's life and allows her to remain more positive, even if she is well aware of the possibility of recurrence.

Coping with cancer

Every person has a unique tool box of coping strategies that have been accumulated over a lifetime. Most will find what they need to cope with cancer. Seeking information, maintaining hope, turning to family and friends for support, developing a partnership with the health care team and learning stress management techniques are all ways to develop the coping mindset. Many women take this time as an opportunity to learn new coping strategies from health care professionals and other women that can help them and their families cope with this new experience.

Seeking information

Appropriate information can help to allay much of the anxiety and fear associated with the unknown. The type and amount varies with the needs of the woman and her family. Generally, people want to know about diagnostic tests, treatment plan (purpose, expected results, side effects, length of time and scheduling), and prognosis.

Essential but often neglected information concerns how the disease and treatment are likely to affect the person's daily life and work. Your cancer center and support groups provide this kind of help. There are booklets, seminars, stress management training programs and self-help groups for individuals with cancer and their families.

Of course, the health care team is a critical provider of information pertinent to your particular problem. When attending appointments, ask questions. Prepare a list; otherwise, you may forget important points that you have been wondering about. Write down the answers and, ideally, take someone along to help you remember what was said. One can be in a daze during the early phase of diagnosis and treatment so having an extra person to listen and clearly recall is very helpful (see Chapter 17).

Telling others

In most cases, your family and close friends will learn sooner or later that you have cancer. It is usually best to disclose the information yourself, according to your own schedule. Confiding fears and hopes is an important part of developing the coping mindset and, in the long run, it is easier than trying to conceal these important feelings.

Telling young children that their mother has cancer can be especially painful. A woman usually feels tremendous anxiety about how best to inform and explain to children when she is trying to cope herself. Most women are worried about being able to care for their children during treatment and about whether they will be around to help them grow up. The goal in telling children is to give them opportunities to ask questions about the disease and to express their feelings about it. While we all wish to shield our children from bad news, it is better that they experience pain in a way that they understand and can talk about with their parents. Coping with sorrow on their own in forms that become embellished by their imagination is far less reassuring than open discussion with their family. Moreover, if children are not told what is happening, they may become confused and hurt and mistakenly believe that they are responsible. They may also imagine things that are not true. They need to hear what is happening in real language from their parents to be reassured that they are included and respected. There are several excellent books available which can help you explain cancer to children of various ages (see Additional Reading). Also, there may be support groups for children at your cancer center.

Support groups

In most cities and towns there are support groups consisting of people with cancer and trained professionals or volunteers who manage the sessions. The session leader provides a forum where the person with cancer can be open about her thoughts and feelings, and can discover that these are normal and acceptable. Other members of the group often suggest alternative ways to deal with difficult issues, ways that have helped them. Seeing others who are coping with similar situations can help you identify solutions to problems which seem overwhelming initially. In addition, membership in a formal group may help you overcome a feeling of helplessness because you will be offering assistance to others. Support groups can also provide information. As the group participants learn about their disease they may approach problems and find solutions in different ways. Many women find sharing their experiences with others to be helpful.

A word of caution about support groups

Participating in a support group requires an investment in time and energy that may compete with family or other activities. You may experience unexpected emotions in some group sessions. For example, you could be upset by the beliefs or coping mechanisms of other group members. Some groups may not be led by appropriate individuals with reliable skills or information, and unintended emotional consequences could result. If you feel uncomfortable or something does not feel right about any particular group, it is best to leave immediately and seek another group.

Breast Cancer Visitors

In addition to formal support groups, most women will benefit from meeting with a 'survivor.' The Breast Cancer Visitors program of the Cancer Society is a valuable resource to the woman with a new diagnosis of breast cancer. Ideally, this contact should occur while the woman is considering surgery or still in hospital.

The visitors have "been there", and they provide information about living with breast cancer; from finding inner strength, to talking to family and friends, to buying a bathing suit with suitable support. They also offer a 'shoulder to cry on'.

You do not need to wait for a referral from a doctor or nurse to initiate a Breast Cancer Visitors visit. Any woman (or her family and friends) can call the Cancer Society to request a visit either before surgery, during the hospital stay, or afterwards.

Developing a partnership with the health care team

At one time, patients and families were considered to be silent members of the health care team, if indeed they were considered members at all. Today, people with cancer are encouraged to take an active role in treatment planning.

Find out who the players are

The first step in developing a partnership with the health care team is to know who the players are and what each one has to offer. This can be a challenging task as, over time, there are often many different specialists involved in the care of the patient and family. Try to identify one team member who will serve as the leader or navigator: often the family doctor, the oncologist (cancer specialist) or a specialist nurse. It doesn't matter who assumes the role as long as he or she is able to relate to you and your family and will be there for the duration. This person should be available at regular intervals, or when required, to listen to concerns, to direct questions to the appropriate professionals, and as a guide and support (Chapter 17).

Participate in decision-making about treatment

No matter how complex your problem may seem, your health care team members should be able to help you participate in the decision-making process by providing you with understandable information and the framework of the 'big picture'. Once a few of the initial choices are made, you will have time to seek additional resources. The educational process continues through the cancer journey.

Participating in decision-making involves listening to the options, identifying their advantages and disadvantages, and comparing them with you family's and especially your own values and aspirations. Some women want to discuss all of the options, perhaps seeking a second opinion before making an informed decision with or without their families. Others might be uncomfortable making the final decision, but can still participate by clarifying their values and wishes so that the final recommendations for treatment are tailored to their needs. Ask questions so that you make an informed decision you are comfortable with.

Participate in treatment planning

Participation in the treatment planning includes: managing the side effects of the treatment, reporting changes in condition, attending follow-up appointments, providing team members with feedback about how things are progressing, and using the services and supports that are available.

When friends don't call

Lost and strained friendships can be a particularly painful aspect of dealing with cancer. Friends may not call for a variety of reasons. For most, it is because they feel that they will have so little to say that will help, and they fear that instead they might say something hurtful or disturb you when you want to rest. Others are afraid that they will not be able to respond appropriately to your change of appearance, or they are fearful of facing the possibility of your death and the eventuality of their own.

If you believe it is discomfort that is keeping a particular friend from visiting, you might try a phone call to dissolve the barrier. This often reassures them that you are still the same person that they liked before, and that you understand their difficulty. However, don't expect to change or enlighten everyone. We all have our own emotional capabilities and some people cannot be comforted enough to help them maintain the same relationship. You will find that different friends will provide support in different ways at various times, and you will also make new friends along the way who are participating in the same treatment process.

Sexuality

Sexuality need not be affected by the diagnosis of breast cancer but it often is. Many women feel damaged by the surgery and uncomfortable with their bodies. Also, treatment can cause fatigue and other symptoms that decrease desire. The onset of treatment-induced menopause may make intercourse uncomfortable due to vaginal dryness. This can be treated.

The whole process of the diagnosis and treatment may make a woman less interested in sex. Her focus may shift to other issues or she might feel depressed. This is normal and needs to be openly discussed with her partner. Her partner may also be frightened about losing and/or hurting her. A common myth is that cancer could be contagious. This is entirely false.

By recognizing changes and seeking counseling if necessary, these feelings may improve with time and understanding. Be assured that a satisfying sexual relationship is possible after breast cancer but may take time to establish.

Maintaining hope

Hope is a crucial tool for people with cancer and their families. It is the internal resource that permits one to cope with the stresses associated with diagnosis and treatment. Loss of hope reduces one's ability to adjust to the situation.

Hope means different things to different people, and tends to change over time depending on the stage of the disease and treatment.

Maintaining and nurturing hope is a strategy that can allay anxiety, depression and fear. Nurturing hope means focusing on the present and what is immediately ahead, rather than on the future or the past, neither of which can be changed. While this reorientation of focus can be difficult, it can help you manage the daily challenges of cancer treatment.

Hope can be affected by the behavior of others. Family members and friends can support the idea that being hopeful is a good thing, and they should not classify hope as being false.

'Be prepared for the worst but hope for the best. There is no such thing as false hope. Every day I hope for a miracle, but that doesn't stop me from continuing my treatment nor would it stop me from acceptance if my treatment is no longer working. If you took my hope away, I don't know if I would want to continue...'

Hope is not based on false optimism or benign reassurance, but is built on the belief that better days or moments can come in spite of the situation.

How can friends and family help you cope with breast cancer?

Practical support

While loved ones may feel powerless to help you with the cancer, they are eager to do something practical or tangible to lighten your load. Practical help is very important during breast cancer treatments and this help comes in many forms. For example, one thoughtful person organized a 'meals on wheels' for her friend during her radiation treatment. Another woman vividly recalled how her elderly father got up nightly to feed her four month old son so that she could rest longer.

Ask friends or family members to take you to your chemotherapy and radiation treatments and clinic appointments in order to be that extra listener. You could also ask them to bring over your favorite food or to do the grocery shopping or the laundry. Let them clean the house, mow the lawn and look after the car. They could help with child care. Accept their offers to take you to a humorous movie or play.

You could go wig and hat shopping with a friend. Or ask for hats as gifts, instead of flowers. Of course, flowers are nice too, as is the occasional box of chocolates! Get your friends to help you with holiday preparations. During treatments, you may be too tired to write Christmas cards or thank-you notes. If you want to send cards and notes, your friends or relatives could help you write them.

Single women living alone report welcoming daily telephone calls from friends and family. These women also sometimes appreciate friends or family spending nights with them, especially when they were feeling particularly ill or vulnerable. A daughter might move home to be with her mother, or a sister might move in during treatment.

Emotional support

People sometimes appreciate being listened to unconditionally, especially when they need to rant and rave or feel sorry for themselves. We all need someone with whom we can do that. Friends and family members who are not afraid to talk about breast cancer are helpful. If the woman feels her friends or family members are not able to hear these things, she may spend a lot of time reassuring them that she is fine, although she may suffer from being unable to unburden herself.

Many women want to be hugged, especially when the tears are flowing.

Some draw strength from frequent phone calls and visits. Many enjoy going for walks with friends. Receiving letters and cards can be welcome and reassuring. Humor is often appreciated.

Friends and relatives also need to know when to leave you in peace. Sometimes the visits and support become 'too much'. It can be tiring if you feel a need to entertain friends and relatives when they visit. To balance a desire for support with the need for time alone, a case manager could coordinate your friends' efforts to be helpful. Otherwise, it is important for you to be forthright and others should understand.

You may experience mixed feelings about self-help books, motivational tapes, megavitamin diets or herbal remedies offered with the best of intentions by friends and relatives. Some women appreciate this type of advice and muster the energy to take it to heart. For others, gifts that possibly imply that one is somehow responsible for their disease only makes them feel angry or guilty.

Many women resent advice to think positively wondering if the implication is that if she had been a positive thinker, she would not have breast cancer. Relatives and friends have to bear in mind that it is may be difficult to think positively, let alone get out of bed in the morning, when you're exhausted by your treatment.

Vulnerable times

The weekend before your first treatments can be a very anxiety-ridden time for you. That's when it's important for your friends and family to rally round and listen to your fears or help you with practical chores.

You may also have a difficult time when your breast cancer treatments come to an end. Suddenly, you will no longer be under the intense scrutiny of your health-care providers and you may feel somewhat abandoned. Your ongoing fears of the cancer returning may escalate at this time, especially since you are no longer actively fighting the disease with therapy. Your family and friends need to be made aware of these fears so that they can support you. Breast cancer is a frightening disease that can undermine you on every front. However, sympathetic relatives and friends can help you in your fight against this disease and, as one woman reported, "help you get your life back".

CHAPTER THIRTY-THREE

Physical therapy and management of lymphedema

MANY BREAST CANCER TREATMENTS such as surgery, radiation and chemotherapy have side effects that can be reduced or eliminated by physical therapy. Preventing physical limitations can help restore and maintain your overall health and fitness and enhance your quality of life.

Exercise during and after surgery and radiation therapy

Most women with breast cancer have two types of surgery. One removes the tumor from the breast (lumpectomy or mastectomy) and the second, axillary dissection, is done to determine whether the breast cancer has spread to the lymph nodes underneath the arm (see Chapter 19). Axillary dissection may lead to difficulties in shoulder motion and weakness, and can contribute to lymphedema or arm swelling.

After any type of surgery, one can expect some pain, discomfort, stiffness and swelling. This is especially true after axillary dissection. Up to 50% of women who undergo this procedure develop tightness, pain, and the formation of 'cords' in the armpit, inner elbow and wrist within a few weeks after their surgery. These thin, visible cords are the hardened lymphatic vessels which have been interrupted by the removal of axillary lymph nodes. Some reduction in the range of arm motion may occur temporarily due to cording. Usually, within several weeks, the cords will rupture on their own and arm motion will return. Radiation therapy may also increase the stiffness in the chest and shoulder muscles. Some women require physical therapy to return to their pre-surgical levels of shoulder motion and upper body strength.

Exercise during and after chemotherapy

Chemotherapy may also make you feel tired. Although it is important to get extra rest, you may feel better if you maintain or improve your overall fitness by exercising three to five days per week. Chemotherapy can also cause joint pain or stiffness similar to arthritis-like pains. Specific types of regular exercise that are gentle on your joints, such as walking or swimming or riding a stationary bicycle, may help during this period. Moist heat such as hot packs or a warm bath can help ease joint and muscle aches. Also, cold packs can help reduce acute (sudden) joint pain or swelling.

Exercises to regain the range of shoulder motion after surgery

An important problem to tackle after surgery is to regain full shoulder motion. Some women regain full motion within days after their surgery, but many women have trouble. This is seen especially when trying to: 1) lift your arm forward in front of your face (shoulder flexion), 2) raise your arm out and up at the side (shoulder abduction), and 3) bring your arm behind your back to fasten a bra (shoulder internal rotation). The following exercises can help you regain these motions. The exercises should be started gently when the drain, if any, is removed. This will usually be within the first week after surgery. Exercise may progress to more active stretching by the second week. Doing these exercises will not 'break' anything, nor will they harm the healing process following surgery.

The first two exercises should be done while lying on your back on the floor. In the first exercise (Figure 24), use a broomstick or cane to have the uninvolved arm 'help' stretch the involved arm into the full range of shoulder flexion. Stretch slowly, as far as you can comfortably go, exerting a prolonged pull on the affected arm. In the second floor exercise (Figure 25), put your hands underneath your head and slowly bring both elbows down to the floor. Breathe out as you stretch and try to get your elbows to touch the floor.

191

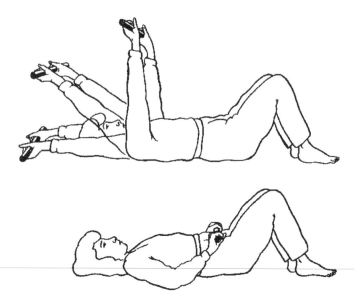

Figure 24: Holding a broomstick helps the unaffected arm stretch the affected arm in this exercise. (Figures 24 to 30 used with permission from Recovering from breast surgery: exercises to strengthen your body and relieve pain. Diane Stumm, Hunter House, 1995.)

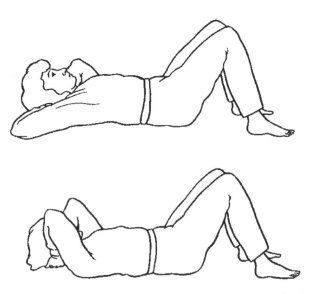

Figure 25: With hands behind your head, elbows are slowly brought down to the floor.

Then relax and breathe in. Breathe out again as you try to stretch a bit further. Repeat each of these exercises four to five times, making sure that your stretches are slow, steady and prolonged.

The third shoulder stretching exercise (Figure 26A) is performed while sitting in a chair or on the floor. It helps to do this exercise in front of a mirror. Once again, use a slow, steady and prolonged stretch to pull your affected arm up over your head and toward your ear. After each stretch, lower your arms and relax. Repeat the stretch four to five times. Once you can do this comfortably, you can increase the pull by bending your trunk sideways toward the side opposite to the involved arm (Figure 26B).

The next two exercises will improve shoulder flexion. Stand facing a wall, with your feet about six inches away from the wall (Figure 27). Try to 'walk' the fingers of both hands up the wall while standing in place. When you have gone as high as you can comfortably go (while feeling a slow, prolonged stretch to your underarm muscles), hold that position for five to 10 seconds to maintain the stretch. To gauge your progress, put a pencil mark at the furthest point to which you can 'walk' your affected arm.

Another shoulder flexion stretch (Figure 28) is done while you are on your hands and knees on the floor. With your hands directly underneath your shoulders and with your knees about 10 to 12 inches apart, slowly lean back on your feet and lower your head to

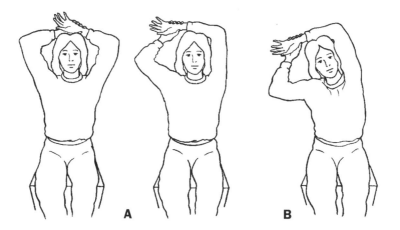

Figure 26: The affected arm is slowly and steadily stretched over your head.

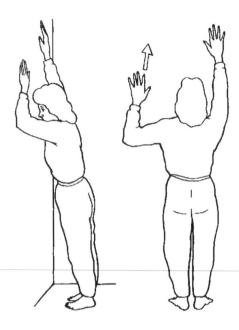

Figure 27: 'Walk' your fingers slowly up the wall, and then the stretch for a few seconds.

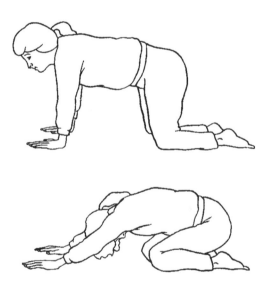

Figure 28: Slowly lean back on your feet and, with elbows straight, lower your head to the floor.

the floor. Keep your elbows straight and feel the pull in your under-arm area. Hold the stretch for five to 10 seconds and then return to the hands-and-knees position. Repeat the stretch four to five times.

Strengthening exercises

It used to be said that vigorous exercises should not be done after breast and axillary surgery. This is no longer true. Once you have full shoulder range of motion, at four to eight weeks after surgery, you can begin to add exercises to increase upper body strength. In the stretching exercise shown in Figure 24, for example, you can add a 1 to 2 pound (½ to 1 kg) weight in each hand and alternately stretch each arm up over your shoulder to strengthen the shoulder muscles. To create your own 1 pound weight, fill a small plastic detergent bottle with sand or pebbles. Or, you can hang a weighted bean bag (2 to 3 pound) over the broom handle or cane and use this to assist in strengthening.

Because the chest muscles are often weakened, especially if you have had a mastectomy, you can strengthen these muscles by doing push-ups while standing against a wall (Figure 29) or from

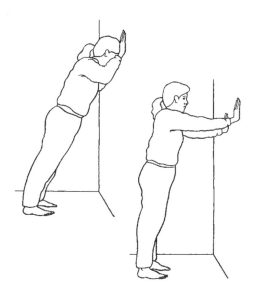

Figure 29: With feet away from the wall, bend your elbows and bring your forehead to the wall. Remember to keep your back straight.

a hands-and-knees position (Figure 30). First, stand with your feet about 2 feet (1/2 meter) apart. Place your hands on the wall, slightly outstretched, at the level of your head. Lean forward to touch your forehead against the wall. Push away slowly until your arms are fully extended. Repeat 8 to 12 times. To make the exercise harder, move your feet back further away from the wall.

The second type of push-up is from a hands-and-knees position (Figure 30). With your knees slightly apart and your hands placed slightly wider than your shoulders, lower your head until your nose touches the floor. Then, straighten your elbows until your arms are fully extended. Repeat 8 to 12 times.

If you had an axillary dissection

Because your lymphatic system has been interrupted as a result of the axillary dissection, it may be advisable to wear a compression

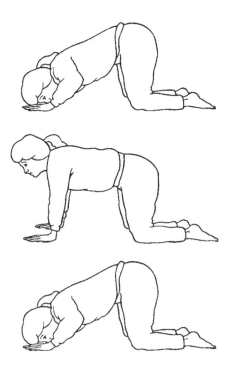

Figure 30: With knees slightly apart and hands wider than your shoulders, do a push-up, lowering your head until it touches the floor.

sleeve on your affected arm when doing weight-training involving more than 10 to 15 pounds (or any other strenuous upper body exercises). This is especially true if using weight-lifting equipment. When using weight machines such as a bench press or latissimus pull-down, start with the smallest weight possible (10 pounds) and increase very gradually. The greatest benefit is derived from weight-training if it is done at least twice a week with a minimum of 8 to 12 repetitions of each exercise.

Aerobic or conditioning exercises for cardiovascular fitness

Overall heart and lung fitness is important to promote health at any age or at any time in your life. Regular aerobic exercise, which increases your heart and breathing rate, can promote a good night's sleep, improve your overall sense of well-being, assist in maintaining ideal body weight and keep your heart and lungs working effectively.

For maximum benefit, you should exercise continuously for 20 to 60 minutes per session, at least three to five days a week. Activities that involve large muscle groups, such as brisk walking, jogging, swimming, cycling, rowing or skating have the greatest benefit.

If you have not done regular exercise before, start out slowly, but commit yourself to doing it regularly. For example, walk four times around a quarter-mile track at your local high school and time yourself. If you don't like walking on a track, use your car to measure the distance of a pleasant walk through your neighborhood. Or, walking on a treadmill in a community center allows you to time your walking speed and measure the distance walked. Continue to walk one mile, three to five times a week, but try to gradually increase your speed over several weeks. However, it is more important to get into a regular habit of walking than to increase your speed. When you can walk a mile in 15 or 16 minutes, increase your distance to one and a half miles.

After menopause a woman loses the protective benefit of estrogens for the bones. As well, chemotherapy and hormonal therapies may further affect the bones and increase the risk of osteoporosis. Therefore, strengthening and weight-bearing exercises to increase bone density are particularly important. A physical therapist or an exercise specialist can suggest a conditioning program for you.

Lymphedema

Women who have had axillary dissection can develop lymphedema (swelling) in the affected arm. Lymphedema occurs because the lymph fluid, which bathes the tissues in your arm to keep them free of infections, can no longer leave the arm through its normal channels in your armpit because they were disrupted by treatment. About 5% to 20% of women who have had axillary dissection will develop permanent lymphedema, usually within two years after their treatment most of which is minor but sometimes can be severe. Some women (7%) develop transient (or temporary) lymphedema which disappears within a few months after breast cancer treatment.

It is therefore important that you report any sensations of puffiness or heaviness in your arm to your physical therapist or doctor. To determine if lymphedema is present, you should have the circumference of both your arms measured. It is recommended that measurements be made using a tape measure at four specific points on your arm: at the mid-palm of the hand, wrist, and 10 cm below and 15 cm above the elbow. Any single measurement that is longer on the affected side by 2 cm or more is considered to be significant lymphedema and requires treatment.

Treating lymphedema

If you develop lymphedema you will need help from physicians, physical therapists, nurses, massage therapists and, sometimes psychosocial counselors if the condition of your arm is causing you to be depressed.

For temporary lymphedema, elevation of the arm, a compression sleeve worn with activity, or close monitoring may be all that is required. Permanent lymphedema may require compression therapy, which involves the use of a compression sleeve or pump. Compression pump therapy can be carried out several times a week or as needed. Physical therapists specializing in lymphedema care offer pump therapy and compression garments, as do many cancer centers.

A form of massage to stimulate lymphatic drainage, called manual lymph drainage (MLD) or manual lymph treatment (MLT), is gaining popularity. It involves bandaging and special exercises and is usually carried out by massage therapists. Complex physical therapy (CPT) or complex decongestive therapy (CDP) is a treatment program which combines MLD, bandaging, exercises, support garments, and skin care counseling to control lymphedema.

Lymphedema is easier to control if you are not overweight and if you exercise regularly. It used to be said that if you have lymphedema you shouldn't do active exercise with your arm, such as playing tennis, squash, lifting weights, rowing, or cross-country skiing. However, this is likely wrong. Your arm will certainly let you know which activities worsen the lymphedema. You may want to wear a compression sleeve during vigorous upper body exercise.

Avoid scratches, burns, cuts and bruises to your involved arm. When you need procedures to be done, such as having blood drawn, intravenous lines started or injections given, try to have them done on your healthy arm. Also, injuries can cause swelling or infection which is not handled well by the stagnant lymphatic system in your affected arm. Therefore, always be on the lookout for signs of infection in your arm (painful redness of your skin) and get immediate treatment. The infections are almost always caused by bacteria called streptococci which respond well to penicillin. You should have some antibiotics on hand to be taken at the first sign of infections, especially if you are traveling to a remote area.

Preventing lymphedema

The following are key points for helping to prevent problems from lymphedema if you have had an axillary dissection.

- Try to maintain an ideal body weight because obesity is a risk factor for lymphedema.
- Try to avoid having your blood pressure taken, blood drawn, injections or vaccinations, or intravenous lines started in the involved arm. If you have had bilateral mastectomies, use the arm that did not have lymph nodes removed. If both sides had lymph nodes removed from the armpit, alternate which arm you use.
- Protect your arm from cuts, scratches and infections by wearing an oven mitt rather than using a pot-holder around the stove and oven. Also wear a gardening glove and long sleeves while digging, pruning, planting or berry picking.

- Consider wearing a compression sleeve when lifting heavy weights or engaging in vigorous upper body exercise such as cross-country skiing, rowing or tennis. It used to be thought that you shouldn't do active exercise, but that advice has changed in recent years.
- Report any signs of arm swelling, pain or redness or any suggestion of infection to your health-care provider immediately.
- Some women wear a compression sleeve when they fly, particularly on a long flight. There is no compelling evidence to show this is of benefit but if you have had problems with arm swelling after an airplane flight it may be worthwhile considering.

CHAPTER THIRTY-FOUR

Reconstructive surgery

Should I or shouldn't I?

NOT ALL WOMEN ARE INTERESTED in breast reconstruction. Some feel that the cancer operation itself is quite enough. Others will opt for additional surgery to reconstruct the breast. It is a personal decision and no particular way is "right". The most common reason for breast reconstruction is the psychological desire to feel 'whole' again. The goal is to restore self-image and self-confidence and improve quality of life.

Women seeking breast reconstruction need to be physically and mentally healthy, must understand the associated risks and complications, and be motivated from within. They should not be undertaking reconstruction to please others in their lives. Occasionally, a patient's poor health or poor prognosis from their disease means that they cannot be considered for this operation. Also, some women are emotionally unprepared to undergo further surgery, with its related risks and potential complications.

Breast cancer treatment always takes precedence

Breast reconstruction should not interfere with the treatment of the patient's breast cancer. The breast cancer surgeon, plastic surgeon and oncologist should ensure that the plans for reconstruction are integrated into the cancer treatment program. Reconstruction generally does not interfere with detection of possible recurrence of the cancer on the chest or elsewhere in the body.

The first visit to the plastic surgeon

The initial referral to a plastic surgeon is usually arranged by the patient's breast surgeon, family physician or her oncologist. The patient will be asked questions about her expectations, desires, and general health, and a brief physical examination will be done. The available reconstructive options will be discussed and the preferred option for the individual patient will be explained in greater detail. The patient should ask questions about the options available, details of the surgical procedure, the degree of pain, the recovery time and the risks. She should expect the surgeon to provide diagrams and photographs or introductions to other patients so that she acquires a realistic sense of the possible results and what to expect during the postoperative recovery period. While every surgeon has produced excellent results, breast reconstruction is not an exact science and possible postoperative complications and patient factors may contribute to a result that falls somewhat short.

Factors that affect the choice of reconstructive procedure

Reconstruction is designed to correct surgical changes. The type of procedure recommended will depend on the type and extent of the surgery (see Chapter 19), but other factors also influence the choice of procedure and the expected cosmetic result. These will differ from one woman to another and include the amount and looseness of the skin, direction and length of the original surgical scar, the amount of fat under the skin, the possibility of skin changes caused by radiotherapy, and the shape and size of the other breast. An additional factor relates to the timing of the reconstructive surgery. Surgery can be done at the time of mastectomy (immediate reconstruction) or at some time following recovery (delayed reconstruction). The choice of method will depend on the combination of the woman's wishes, the surgeon's and oncologist's preference, the type and extent of the cancer operation, and the nature of the opposite breast.

Surgical techniques

Tissue expanders and implants

A tissue expander is a device that looks like an empty plastic bag with an attached valve. It is surgically placed behind the pectoralis muscle. In the weeks following surgery, the expander is inflated using a small amount of saline (salt water). The idea is that after the surgical site has healed, the bag can be enlarged gradually by injecting salt water into the valve every one to two weeks. Like the abdominal skin during pregnancy, the skin of the chest will stretch as the 'pseudo-breast' enlarges. Usually, this process goes on for several months in order to overstretch the skin to a size larger than the normal breast. Then, a second operation is done to remove the expander and replace it with a permanent breast implant (Figure 31).

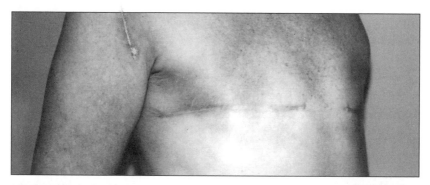

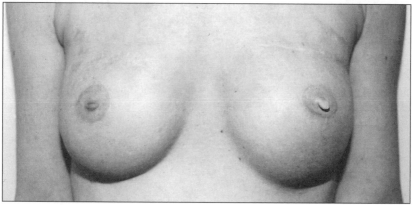

Figure 31: The result of breast and nipple reconstruction of both breasts. Tissue expanders were used to stretch the skin from the preoperative stage (upper) until there was sufficient room for the implants to be inserted. At a later operation the nipples were reconstructed (lower).

An 'implant' is a fluid or silicone-filled bag shaped like a small round or oval cushion. The implant is typically placed through a portion of the old incision, against the ribs, tucked underneath the pectoralis muscle. The surgery is done under general anesthetic and usually involves a brief hospitalization. Postoperatively, there may be drains in place to remove any fluid build-up, and there will often be more pain than from the original mastectomy.

Most often, reconstruction involves a 2-step procedure: insertion of the tissue expander and later, removal of the expander and insertion of the implant. Occasionally there is enough skin and normal tissue remaining after the mastectomy that an implant can be inserted directly. The use of a tissue expander is appropriate when there is not enough skin remaining to allow insertion of an implant large enough to match the volume or shape of the other breast. Many surgeons who use tissue expanders believe that by overstretching the skin, there will be a more natural droop to the breast after placement of the permanent implant.

Complications of implant reconstruction include infection, bleeding or problems related to the implant itself, such as the development of a layer of scar tissue around the implant. This scar tissue forms a fibrous 'capsule' around the implant that may contract and squeeze the implant into a firm, round ball. This is called 'capsular contracture'. If this happens the implant will feel firm and will retract up the chest wall. This may be unsightly and uncomfortable and may require more surgery to correct it. When radiation is used before or after an implant-type reconstruction, approximately 50% of patients will develop capsular contracture. The chance of developing capsular contracture in the absence of previous radiation is approximately 10% to 20%.

The most common disadvantage of the tissue expander—implant form of reconstruction is failure to achieve a shape similar to the opposite breast. Another disadvantage is that it involves two operations (as do most breast reconstructions) and extra visits to a doctor's office for the fluid injections. In addition, saline (salt water filled) implants may leak and deflate. If this occurs, more surgery will be required to replace the implant with a new one.

Over the past decade, textured saline implants and tissue expanders have been introduced in the hope of decreasing the risk of capsular contracture and optimizing the shape of the reconstructed breast. However, there is a tendency for these devices to become relatively immobile on the chest wall and patient satisfaction with the textured saline implants has been low except in patients in whom reconstruction of both breasts is required.

Myocutaneous flaps

Myocutaneous flaps involve shifting a piece of tissue that includes skin, fat and muscle from one part of the body to another. Often, a portion of the flap remains attached to its original site to ensure that the tissue in the flap has an adequate blood supply. The rationale for the use of myocutaneous flaps is that by using the body's own tissue, a more natural-feeling breast may be created, avoiding the complications related to implants. However, there is a trade-off, since the more complex surgery involves increased risks, scarring, potential donor site problems and increased recovery time.

In one type of myocutaneous flap operation, the latissimus dorsi muscle (the large triangular muscle from the back) along with the overlying skin is moved into the mastectomy area. For some women, enough tissue can be transferred from the back to create a good breast size (medium B cup). If a larger breast is required, this procedure can be combined with a small implant to optimize volume. However, this operation leaves a scar and a contour deformity on the back and elim-inates the latissimus as a functioning muscle in the back (Figure 32). Surprisingly, most patients are not aware of this lost function after-wards. The hospital stay is approximately two to three days. Often, the patient is discharged with a drain in the back donor site and will require home care until this is removed.

Currently, the most commonly used flap technique is the 'Transverse Rectus Abdominus Muscle' flap, know as the TRAM flap. Of all the options, this type of surgery will produce the best results for those patients who are highly motivated, have a suitable abdomen, and are willing to tolerate a longer recovery phase. This method uses a large section of skin and fat from the lower abdomen (belly) along with a portion of one of the rectus (sit-up) muscles which provides the blood supply to the tissue. A breast mound is fashioned out of the skin and fat which has been brought up from the abdomen (Figure 33).

The abdominal defect from where the muscle is taken (donor site) is repaired with sutures, and sometimes requires reinforce-ment with surgical mesh. Postoperatively, the patient is mobilized slowly and typically spends four days in hospital. The abdominal

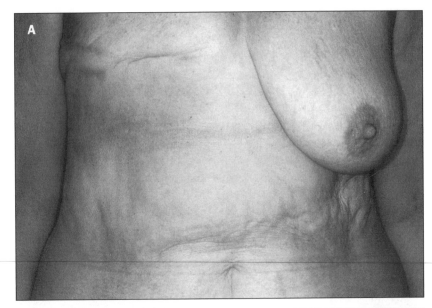

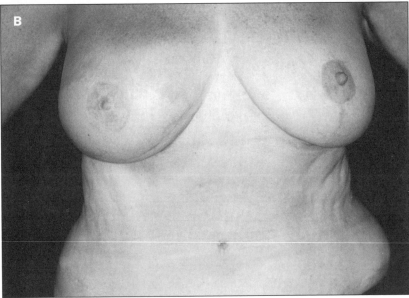

Figure 32: Preoperative (32A) and one year postoperative (32B) appearance of a woman with a delayed TRAM flap reconstruction and left reduction mammoplasty carried out for symmetry. The abdominal scar is just visible above the panty line. At a second operation the right-sided nipple was created.

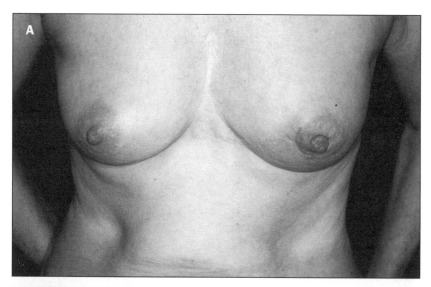

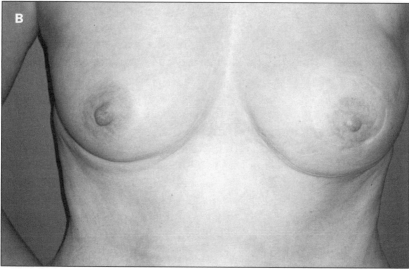

Figure 33: Preoperative (33A) and one year postoperative (33B) comparison of a woman who had an immediate TRAM flap reconstruction of the left breast. A skin-sparing mastectomy was done through the small circular scar surrounding the left areola in 33B, and the patient's own nipple and areola was removed along with the underlying breast tissue. The breast mound is composed of tissue transferred from the site of the new abdominal scar. In a second-stage operation, the nipple and areola in 33B were fashioned surgically and with tattooing.

area is more uncomfortable than the chest as a result of muscle spasms. Drains will be present at the breast site as well as in the abdomen donor site, and will gradually be removed as the amount of drainage decreases. Recovery time is usually six to 12 weeks, depending on the patient. Strenuous abdominal activity is discouraged for six to eight weeks. The amount of time off work averages six to 12 weeks; however, some patients require more time.

Although using the body's own tissues sounds attractive, this is a complex method of breast reconstruction, with additional possible complications, including abdominal wall hernia (about 2%), part of the flap not surviving (5% to 20% in non-smokers, higher in smokers), thrombophlebitis (formation of blood clots in the veins), healing problems in the abdominal site and postoperative lung problems (rare). If reconstruction is done at the time of mastectomy, there is an increased risk of a portion of the mastectomy flap not surviving in about 10% to 15% of patients. Although this may not ultimately affect the overall reconstructive result, it requires extra wound care and dressings to the area over a period of several weeks.

Women at highest risk for complications are those with large, heavy breasts, diabetics, smokers, those with chronic lung disease, immune arthritic conditions, or those who have had previous radiation therapy to the breast or chest wall. The reason for the added risk is that these conditions affect the adequacy of blood flow into the flap. Good blood flow into the flap is essential to proper healing and function of the flap tissue. These patients should only be considered candidates for flap surgery if the surgeon has extensive experience in these techniques and the patient is extremely motivated and understanding of the potential risks. Most surgeons require patients to quit smoking beforehand, ideally two to three months prior to TRAM flap surgery. Another issue which may prevent the use of a TRAM flap is the presence of other surgical scars in the abdomen which may have disrupted the necessary blood supply to the abdominal tissue.

A side benefit of TRAM flap breast reconstruction is a free 'tummy tuck' (Figure 32). However, if a patient has had a previous tummy tuck procedure, they can no longer be considered for this surgery. Previous abdominal liposuction can also increase the risks associated with the TRAM flap procedure, and may have reduced the available fatty tissue to an inadequate volume for this type of operation.

Second-stage breast reconstruction

Most breast reconstruction should be viewed as a two-staged surgical procedure. The first step is to create a new breast mound using one of the techniques already discussed. The second procedure is planned four to six months later and should be viewed as a minor procedure to optimize symmetry between the two breasts and reconstruct a nipple. If the original reconstruction was a flap procedure, then minor scar revisions are usually done at this time.

Nipple reconstruction

Most women who seek breast reconstruction are happy once a breast mound has been created but, if offered, will opt to have completion of their reconstruction by the creation of a nipple and areola. There are various techniques available to achieve this, and to a large extent the technique selected will depend on the preference and experience of the plastic surgeon. Typically, a projecting nipple can be made from small flaps of tissue raised up locally off the previously created breast mound (Figure 32), or it can be taken from the opposite nipple as a graft if the opposite nipple is large. The more darkly pigmented areola can be fashioned from a portion of the opposite areola or a skin graft from high on the inside of the thigh, or it can simply be tattooed. Nipple-areola reconstruction is relatively minor surgery. The main problems relate to partial graft failure, loss of projection of the reconstructed nipple and mismatched color.

Matching the breast exactly

Paradoxically, the easiest situation for achieving identical-looking breasts (symmetry) with mastectomy reconstruction is when both breasts are reconstructed (Figure 31). When only one breast has had surgery, the goal of reconstruction is to match the normal breast, but an exact match is seldom possible. To get a close match, the normal breast may need to be altered. This may require a breast uplift (mastopexy) or reduction of the normal breast. Both of these procedures create some scars on the normal breast, and introduce some risks and potential complications. Despite this, symmetry surgery of the opposite breast is generally very well tolerated and often gives the patient a more youthful, less heavy and droopy breast that more closely matches the reconstructed breast (Figure 32).

Timing of breast reconstruction

Traditionally, breast reconstruction after mastectomy was delayed for a period of time, often a year, to allow time to complete additional therapies such as radiation and chemotherapy, and to allow the woman to recover mentally and physically from her ordeal before she proceeded with more extensive surgery. Alternatively, the reconstruction procedure may be done at the same time as the mastectomy. Advantages of this include reducing the number of operations and reducing the necessary recovery time and time off work, lessening the body image disturbance and grief reaction that many patients suffer after mastectomy, and optimizing the overall cosmetic result by allowing a skin-sparing (skin-saving) mastectomy (Figure 33). However, despite the improved cosmetic results that are often attainable with immediate reconstruction, patients in this group are often less satisfied with their reconstruction result compared to those who have had to live with a mastectomy deformity for a period of time prior to reconstruction.

Disadvantages of immediate reconstruction include the coordination of two surgeons, a longer operation, and a potentially increased number of complications. Some oncologists prefer that if additional therapies such as chemotherapy and radiation are going to be necessary and the patient is at high risk for wound healing complications (smokers, diabetics, obese patients, large-breasted patients), that reconstruction be done as a delayed rather than immediate procedure. Timing of reconstruction, then, is a decision that should be made in consultation with the patient, the oncologic surgeon and an oncologist involved in the patient's care.

Life-style issues

CHAPTER THIRTY-FIVE

Nutrition

WE EAT TO SATISFY A COMPLEX SET OF NEEDS—emotional, cultural, sensual and of course, nutritional. Eating well, in every sense of the word, is one of the most supportive things that a woman with breast cancer can do for herself.

What is a healthy diet?

A healthy diet includes a wide variety of whole grain cereals and breads, vegetables, fruit, legumes (beans), lentils, nuts and seeds as well as lean meat, chicken, fish and low-fat dairy products or other high-calcium foods. Balance is also important to achieve adequate essential nutrients such as protein, vitamins, minerals and fiber. The Healthy Eating Plan is recommended as a guideline. This plan can be used by women with a variety of food preferences, including those who eat a vegetarian diet. Vegetarians should choose legumes (beans), lentils, nuts and seeds from the 'Meat and Alternatives' group, and select a variety of calcium-rich foods daily.

Is there a link between diet and breast cancer?

Among other factors, diet may influence the risk of developing breast cancer. However, the importance of diet in comparison to other more established risk factors such as reproductive and genetic factors is unknown. Certainly, many women who eat healthy diets can, and do, develop breast cancer.

Nevertheless, the consumption of alcohol, high in fat diets and limited use of fruits and vegetables may increase the risk of developing breast cancer. In addition, being overweight may also raise the risk of developing breast cancer. At present, several large, long-term studies are in progress to determine whether women who follow low-fat diets are less likely to develop breast cancer. There is also interest in whether diets rich in fruits, vegetables, whole grains, and legumes may be protective.

The benefits of a good diet after diagnosis of breast cancer

Once you have had breast cancer, changing your diet may be beneficial. Eating foods low in fat and rich in vitamins, minerals, fiber and protective compounds found in plant foods may reduce the risk of breast cancer recurrence. Achieving and maintaining a healthy body weight is also important, and is more easily achieved on a lower calorie plant-based diet. Studies are being conducted to determine whether diet can delay or reduce the risk of breast cancer recurrence in women who have completed cancer treatment(s). Results of these long term studies are expected within the next few years.

A healthy diet following breast cancer is also important for maintaining general well-being, and for preventing a variety of other health conditions such as heart disease, diabetes, osteoporosis and obesity.

Is there a special diet to follow during cancer treatment?

Your body needs a wide variety of nutrients to aid in healing after surgery or while undergoing radiation therapy or chemotherapy. The Healthy Eating Plan can be used as a guide to select foods during treatment and recovery.

However, treatment for breast cancer or a recurrence can cause side effects that at times make eating more difficult. Some women experience nausea, vomiting, weight changes, diarrhea (or constipation), a sore mouth or throat, a change in appetite, or a change in the way food tastes. Almost all women will experience fatigue. Modifications to your diet, along with a 'once-a-day' multivitamin/mineral supplement, may be recommended if you are unable to eat a variety of vegetables, fruits and whole grain foods.

If you are having chemotherapy

During chemotherapy, nausea, a sore mouth, taste changes and mild diarrhea may occur.

Ease nausea with starchy snacks and light drinks

Nausea is best controlled by a combination of medications and certain foods. Dry, starchy foods like crackers and dry cereals, eaten often, help minimize the 'empty stomach' feeling that can make nausea worse.

Fluids like flat ginger ale, weak tea, diluted fruit juice or ice water are generally better tolerated than milkshakes, coffee or very sweet juices. Keeping a thermos or large cup close by can help remind you of the importance of drinking lots of fluid during chemotherapy.

If the smell of cooking food makes nausea worse, try to avoid being in the kitchen. If this is not realistic, consider purchased or homemade meals that can be easily reheated.

Soothe mouth sores

If mouth sores occur during chemotherapy, certain foods such as oranges and grapefruit, salty or spicy foods, or rough foods, like toast, should be avoided until the sores heal. Many women find cold foods like fruit, yogurt, ice milk and blended shakes very soothing.

If foods taste different

Some women notice that certain foods taste different during chemotherapy. For example, meat might taste bitter or metallic. If this happens, high-protein alternatives such as eggs, milk or tofu will make eating more enjoyable. Food cravings can also occur. Some women crave 'comfort foods' during treatment, whereas others find that fruit and certain vegetables are the most appealing foods.

Coping with diarrhea and gas

You can minimize diarrhea by limiting your intake of alcohol, strong coffee, strong tea and cola, and by temporarily eating fewer high-fiber foods such as bran cereals and whole grain breads. Excess gas can be at least partially controlled by eating fewer gas-forming foods such as legumes (beans) and vegetables from the cabbage family, such as cabbage, Brussels sprouts and broccoli.

If you are having radiation therapy

During radiation, fatigue and a mild sore throat may occur.

If you are feeling tired

The use of convenience or take-out foods, leftovers or previously prepared and frozen meals can reduce the effort of meal preparation. If possible, arrange to have some meals prepared by family or friends, or use grocery delivery or catering services. As well, simple meals can still be nutritious, for example, a sandwich or a bowl of cereal with milk and fruit.

Sore throat or difficulty swallowing

Women whose radiation treatment involves the throat area sometimes develop temporary soreness or discomfort during swallowing. Eating soft, moist foods is helpful, such as hot or cold cereals, soups, pasta, fruit, yogurt, poached eggs, canned fish, or chicken stew. If needed, a smooth consistency can be achieved by putting foods through a blender. Very hot foods such as tea, soup or spicy foods can make a sore throat worse.

If you are having hormonal therapy

Some hormonal treatments that lower estrogen may cause bone loss and over time increase the risk of osteoporosis. Post-menopausal women and those who experience early menopause due to chemotherapy are at increased risk of bone loss. As a result, adequate calcium (1500 mg) and vitamin D (800 IU) are recommended daily from combined food sources and supplements. Pre-menopausal women require 1200 mg of calcium and 400 IU vitamin D.

What about gaining weight during treatment?

Regardless of the type of treatment you are receiving, weight gain is common in women with breast cancer. It occurs most often in pre-menopausal women treated with chemotherapy and/or hormone therapy. The exact cause of weight gain is unclear, but it could be due to a number of factors including decreased physical activity, eating frequently to control nausea, eating as an antidote to boredom or stress, or because of an increased appetite or food cravings. If you have experienced natural or treatment-related menopause, are taking Megace®, or have recently quit smoking, you may also notice that your weight has increased.

How can weight gain be managed?

Weight loss during treatment may put unnecessary stress on the body, reduce energy levels and delay recovery. Therefore, aim to avoid weight gain and maintain your weight until treatment is completed. You can do this by eating more fruits, vegetables and whole grains, which are low in calories. Reducing the portion size of food and limiting high-fat foods will also help to achieve or maintain a healthy weight. If frequent eating is necessary to control nausea, low-fat foods such as low-fat crackers, cereal with skim milk, bread and jam, and fruit are good choices.

Being more physically active will also promote weight loss and has a number of other health benefits such as improved mood, sleep, body image and increased muscle and bone mass. Your doctor or registered dietitian can offer you more individualized advice.

Are extra vitamins and minerals helpful during treatment?

Despite the popularity and common use of vitamin and mineral supplements, it's not yet clear whether their use helps in cancer treatment. Those who support supplement use suggest that they may restore immune function. Although a number of nutrients are required for the immune system (including vitamins A, C, E, B6, beta-carotene, folic acid, zinc and iron), too much of a good thing is not necessarily better, and can be harmful. For example, too much zinc actually depresses the immune system.

Another popular theory is that the antioxidant vitamins—vitamins C, E, and beta-carotene—are required to help repair cells damaged during cancer treatment. Although foods that are rich in antioxidants (dark green and orange vegetables and a variety of fruits) are recommended as part of a healthy diet, at present there is not enough evidence to indicate that antioxidant supplements are safe and beneficial during cancer treatment. If you are thinking of using vitamin or mineral supplements in high doses during treatment, discuss it with your physician and registered dietitian.

Once treatment is over

Many women notice that they gain weight in the years after a breast cancer diagnosis. Some attribute the weight gain to tamoxifen but in research studies the amount of weight gain has been similar whether women were taking tamoxifen or placebo. The weight gain seems to be related to ageing, reduced metabolism relate to hormonal changes, depression or changes in the woman's priorities regarding food, her health and body image. Ultimately, weight gain or loss is related to an imbalance between the amount of calories eaten and the energy burned off doing the activities of daily living and additional exercise.

If you have completed your cancer treatment and haven't already made healthful changes to your diet, this is the best time to start. Eating less fat and more fruit, vegetables and whole-grain foods can help you regain the sense of control and well-being that will enhance your recovery. Besides a possible connection to breast cancer risk, too much fat in the diet has also been linked to the development of heart disease and obesity. In addition, low-fat diets and those rich in fruits and vegetables are being studied regarding their possible link to the prevention of breast cancer recurrence.

Increasing the emphasis on wholesome and naturally low-fat foods such as whole grains, legumes (beans) and lentils, fruits and vegetables can reduce the fat in your diet. You can also limit fat by removing visible sources on chicken or meat wherever possible, and by using low-fat cooking methods such as poaching, broiling and baking. In addition, use less butter, margarine or mayonnaise on sandwiches and use light salad dressings or extra herbs and spices to flavor food. As you probably know, foods such as crackers, cookies, cakes, potato chips, ice cream and cheese are generally high in fat. Reading food labels to check the amount of fat is a good idea and will help you choose low-fat alternatives. A registered dietitian can provide further advice.

Ongoing research for unanswered questions

Research in the area of diet and breast cancer is constantly evolving in an attempt to answer many remaining questions. For example, it is not yet known whether women who have had breast cancer should include or avoid some specific foods, such as higher-fat foods, alcohol, and soy and flax based foods (which contain plant estrogens). Also, it has not yet been determined whether women with a history of breast cancer will benefit from additional vitamin and minerals supplements. However, healthy eating is always a positive step in general. At this time, The Healthy Eating Plan is a balanced recommendation for women.

More advice on nutrition*

You can obtain further advice about nutrition by contacting a registered dietitian at your regional cancer center or community hospital. As well, in some cities there are nutrition hotlines staffed by qualified dietitians. Check with your local dietetic association about resources in your area.

In the United States, the phone number of the Consumer Nutrition Hotline of the American Dietetic Association is 1-800-366-1655. In B.C., Dial-a-Dietitian can be reached at 1-800-667-DIET.

The Additional Reading section includes cookbooks devoted to lower fat, higher fiber meals. The recipes are easy to follow and, most importantly, taste great!

* See our Healthy Eating Plan on the following page.

Healthy Eating Plan

In one day you should eat:

5 to 12 servings of grain products

5 to 10 servings of vegetables and fruit

2 to 4 servings of milk products

2 to 3 servings of meat and alternatives

Grain products (each is 1 serving)
- 1 slice of bread
- $1/2$ a bagel or pita bread
- $1/2$ cup (125 ml) of cooked pasta or rice
- $3/4$ cup (175 ml) of cooked cereal
- 30 g of dry cereal ($1/3$ to 1 cup, depending on the type of cereal)

Vegetables and fruit (each is 1 serving)
- 1 medium-sized vegetable or fruit, such as one carrot, potato, apple, orange or banana
- $1/2$ cup (125 ml) of vegetables or fruit, such as corn, broccoli, berries, peas, or applesauce
- 1 cup (250 ml) of salad
- $1/2$ cup (125 ml) of juice

Milk products (each is 1 serving)

Milk products are an excellent source of calcium. Each serving contains approximately 300 mg of calcium.
- 1 cup (250 ml) of milk
- $3/4$ cup (175 g) of yogurt
- 2 ounces (50 g) of cheese
- 1 cup (250 ml) fortified soy beverage*

Meat and alternatives (each is 1 serving)
- 2-3 ounces (50–100 g) of lean meat
- $1/3$–$2/3$ can (50–100 g) of tuna or salmon
- $1/2$–1 cup (125–50 ml) cooked legumes, eg. beans, lentils, split peas
- $1/3$ cup (100 g) tofu
- 1–2 eggs
- 2 tablespoons (30 ml) of nut or seed butter
- 3–4 tablespoons (45–60 ml) nuts or seeds

Other Calcium rich foods

$3 1/2$ oz (8 med.) sardines, canned (370 mg)

1 cup (250 ml) calcium fortified orange juice (300 mg)

3 oz (90 g) salmon, canned with bones (180 mg)

1 Tbsp (15 ml) blackstrap molasses (170 mg)

$1/4$ cup (60 ml) almonds (95 mg)

1 medium orange (55 mg)

2 medium figs, dried (54 mg)

$1/2$ cup (125 ml) broccoli (35 mg)

*Fortified soy beverage contains added calcium, vitamins A and D, riboflavin and B12 and is available in some areas.

CHAPTER THIRTY-SIX

Stress and relaxation

What is stress?

STRESS IS WOVEN INTO THE FABRIC OF LIFE. At healthy levels it challenges us and promotes activity, but when you feel 'overloaded' or 'lose control' then the stress is no longer healthy. The uncertainty and fears surrounding a diagnosis of breast cancer can lead to a feeling of overload just when there is a great need to be 'in control' and it can threaten your well-being.

How much stress am I feeling?

Stress is a subjective response that is not expressed the same way in each person. When stress becomes too great, the mind may fool you into thinking that you are 'coping,' but the body gives more accurate signals. If you recognize and acknowledge your own stress response, you is easier to deal with it.

To assess your own response to stress, it is helpful to learn to scan your body while asking yourself questions. Start at the top of your head, searching for tightness between your eyebrows. Are your lips pursed? Is your jaw clenched? Are your shoulders hunched up near your ears? Often, we don't notice these things until we are alerted by a pounding headache or lower back pain at the end of the day. Do you feel a tightness in the throat, a constriction in the chest or a churning stomach? Are you breathing shallowly, using only the upper part of your chest? Does your heart beat fast? Some people notice that their sleep pattern is disturbed, and others eat more than they need because eating is comforting.

When in distress, the mind doesn't focus and function the way it usually does. You may forget your own telephone number or an important appointment. Your thoughts could become dark and repetitive, and after only an hour's sleep you may lie awake for hours doing what has been so aptly called 'awfulizing.' Emotionally, you are not as steady as usual, and find yourself in tears over something that you would normally take in stride.

To be told to 'relax' at a time like this seems unreasonable. However, when you are not feeling the effects of an overload of stress, you find yourself filled with a tranquil energy and a sense of control. How do you achieve this elusive feeling, especially after a recent diagnosis of breast cancer?

How can I reduce stress and regain a sense of control?

Reading this book, gaining knowledge about breast cancer, is one practical way to help you find that sense of control. Also, finding someone to listen, though this sounds simple, is of enormous value.

Research has shown that even twenty minutes a day of relaxation can have a beneficial effect on the body. It doesn't matter whether it is transcendental meditation or simply sitting quietly watching the birds at a feeder outside the window. Twenty minutes of steady walking or other exercise works for some people. Tai-Chi and yoga also use movement to bring the body and mind into a state of harmony. Meditation teaches us to focus our minds on a particular word (mantra) or object (mandala), or on the rising and falling of the breath to still the chattering mind and restore a sense of equilibrium. Anything that allows the body to be at ease and the mind to become quieter brings back balance and harmony. Think of the ocean. Even when a storm is raging, deep below there is a place where the water is calm. So it is with your own self. You need to find the way down to that place deep within yourself where you are calm and in control, even in the midst of chaos.

Women are used to being responsible for others and putting their own needs last. Giving yourself permission to take some time for yourself can be an important part of the healing process. Be your own good care-giver; and know that it is healthy to say 'yes' to your own needs.

The relaxation response

Relaxation is about tranquil energy and gaining a sense of control so that you can respond to situations with good choices. It is interesting that the ancient Chinese symbol for crisis has two components, one meaning 'danger,' the other meaning 'opportunity'. Gaining a sense of control gives you an opportunity to make creative choices.

The breath is the pulse of the mind. You can slow your racing thoughts simply by changing your breathing, especially by breathing from the bottom of the diaphragm instead of the shallow, tight breathing from high in the chest that usually accompanies stress. For example: take a comfortable, deep breath, hold it to the count of four and then let it out with a sigh. Repeat this four times. Feel how your shoulders release and your facial muscles soften. When you find yourself experiencing tension, remind yourself to take a sighing breath.

'Autogenics' is another way to occupy the thinking mind by getting it busy with repeated words such as 'My right arm is heavy, my right arm is warm.' With this repetition, the mind starts to convince the body that its different parts are at ease. This feeling of bodily comfort induces a sense of calm control.

Another way to achieve the relaxation response is to imagine yourself in a beautiful place, perhaps in nature or a delightful room, or to relive the memory of a time of achievement and strength. This is the opposite of 'awfulizing,' as you use your body-mind connection to create sensations of peace and 'connectedness.' Audiotapes can also be very helpful by coaching you through these experiences (see Additional Reading).

'Quick fixes'

Sometimes finding even twenty minutes a day for relaxing seems like a tall order. In this case, experiment with some 'quick fixes' to help familiarize you with the healing benefits of relaxation.

Whenever you are particularly stressed you quite naturally do one of these 'quick fixes' already: you sigh. You can cultivate sighing as a way towards relaxation. After three or four comfortable sighing breaths you will find that the muscles of the face are more at ease, the chest feels more open and the shoulders are softer. Because one needs regular reminders to sigh, try putting little colored dots in all sorts of places such as on your steering wheel, on the telephone or on your purse. These dots can serve as triggers, reminders to take a breath, hold it to the count of four and then sigh the breath out. Do this throughout the day.

Another 'quick fix' is to practice a quick progressive muscle relaxation every time you sit down. Let tension flow from the top of your head out through the soles of your feet. Or take a 30-second vacation and recall a beautiful place or happy, carefree time.

Certain fragrances are known to soothe and elevate one's mood. Try a few drops of neroli oil, lavender, geranium or another fragrance which pleases you as you relax in a warm bath. Many health food stores and pharmacies carry aroma therapy products.

Increasingly, you will recognize the importance of your own role in the healing process in partnership with your physicians and their treatments and medications. Learning your role can add a rich dimension to the power of this partnership.

What if cancer recurs?

CHAPTER THIRTY-SEVEN

Follow-up: Support, side effects and concerns about recurrence

OFTEN, IT IS ONLY AT THE END OF TREATMENT that women start to worry about the possibility of a relapse. 'What if the breast cancer recurs? When will it recur? What can I do to prevent it from coming back? What is my prognosis if it does relapse? Will I die? How long have I got?' Understandably, these disturbing questions can plague the mind.

What are the goals of follow-up?

There are several purposes of regular follow-up after treatment for breast cancer including providing support, to assess, to explain and manage any side effects from treatment and to offer early detection of potentially curable recurrent or new disease. Follow-up visits also give you an opportunity to ask questions and discuss any new information you are wondering about. Unfortunately, although there are many useful treatments should breast cancer recur, there is yet no curative treatment if breast cancer is found in organs beyond the breast and lymph node regions. In follow-up, therefore, the doctors should carefully look for new disease in the breast or lymph nodes. Assessment will include regular mammograms. If a woman has no symptoms, there is no value in doing tests such as chest x-rays, bone scans or blood tests to determine if breast cancer has spread to other organs.

What are the chances of a recurrence?

Recurrences happen because cancer cells were not removed or were resistant to the initial treatment. Recurrence may be 'local' when they occur in the remaining skin, breast, lymph nodes or chest wall, or recurrences may be 'systemic' when they occur in other parts of the body such as the bones, liver or lungs. 'Metastasize' refers to the movement of cancer cells. A new growth in organs beyond the breast is called a 'metastasis.'

The risk of recurrence is related to several factors, including whether the cancer is in situ or invasive, the size of the tumor, and the presence and number of cancer-involved lymph nodes. Patients with only in situ disease have a very low risk of the cancer recurring elsewhere in the body, but there is a possibility of local recurrence in the treated breast or of a cancer developing in the other breast.

For women with invasive cancers, the risk of relapse is related to the clinical stage (Chapter 16). In clinical stage I disease (a small tumor with no cancer found in the axillary lymph nodes), 75% to 95% of patients will be alive with no recurrence 10 years or more after treatment. In more advanced stages, the risk of relapse is greater. Approximately 50% of stage II patients and 75% of those with a stage III cancer will develop a recurrence either locally or elsewhere in the body within 10 years of treatment, if treatment consists of surgery alone.

New therapies for breast cancer are being studied all over the world and the information from these studies is shared internationally in an attempt to improve cure rates. It is hoped that over the next few years fewer women will suffer a relapse.

When should I worry about a new problem?

Most recurrences beyond the breast cause symptoms; they are rarely silent. The symptoms depend on which organ is affected. For example, breast cancer that has traveled to the bones will often cause bone pain, while recurrences in the lungs may cause cough or shortness of breath. It is often difficult for a patient who has recently been diagnosed to know which symptoms might indicate recurrent disease and which symptoms are simply normal aches and pains. It takes time for a woman to start trusting her body again after a diagnosis of breast cancer. Worry about relapse makes it hard to be at ease.

In general, symptoms of recurrence are more persistent than normal aches and pains and become progressively worse. For example, a backache brought on by moving furniture usually feels bad for a day or two and then gradually gets better. Metastatic breast cancer to a bone in the back may come on gradually, may come and go with activity and may respond to pain killers, but it will not go away completely and stay away. Instead, it will become more persistent. If you are worried about a new symptom, especially if it is persistent or getting worse, you should see your doctor. She or he will do an examination and order any necessary investigations. If everything is normal and the symptoms continue to bother you, they could be caused by something other than the breast cancer. Naturally, not all new symptoms mean a recurrence of breast cancer, but your doctor should do an evaluation and arrive at a diagnosis.

How and by whom should I be followed?

All women, after a diagnosis of breast cancer, should have follow-up visits to provide information and support and to check for a local recurrence or metastasis. However, medical opinion differs on the best follow-up schedule, and women's needs also vary. Some women are comfortable with frequent follow-up and the reassurance that there is no detectable recurrence. Other women find that follow-up visits cause unnecessary anxiety. It is important that the woman and her doctor agree on a schedule of follow-up which provides reassurance and support and detects most recurrences promptly, but allows the woman to return to normal living.

It is not essential that you be followed at a cancer center. Many women receive excellent support and surveillance from their family physicians. It is important that you feel confident in the doctor's ability to listen to you and examine you, particularly the treated breast if you have had breast-conserving surgery. If you are seeing several different physicians, space out the visits to avoid duplication.

There is very little advantage to the early detection of recurrence beyond the breast or lymph nodes because currently available treatments for metastatic disease are not curative. Therefore performing lots of x-rays, scans or blood tests to look for metastatic disease are not recommended unless the patient has some new, worrisome symptom that needs to be checked. Local treatment (surgery and/or radiation) may be curative for a local recurrence or a new cancer developing in the opposite breast. Therefore, regular mammograms are the only 'routine' test recommended for a woman who otherwise feels well in the years following breast cancer treatment.

How often should I have follow-up visits and what should happen at the visit?

We recommend a first follow-up visit about six weeks after the treatment (surgery, chemotherapy and radiation therapy) is complete. Then, you should have visits approximately every three to six months for the first three years and then every six to twelve months until year five. After five years, an annual checkup is recommended. At each visit, the physician should ask about your level of appetite, energy, menopausal symptoms, pain, arm swelling and your emotional health. You should expect to be examined, at least in the region of the breasts, arms, neck, chest and abdomen. This visit should also be an opportunity for you to ask questions. Be sure to tell your doctor about any new symptoms or changes in how your body is functioning including aches and pains in bones, a persistent cough or shortness of breath, nausea, weight loss, or new lumps or bumps. Any of these symptoms could possibly be indications of recurrent disease. You should also discuss your psychological and life-style issues and report any menopausal or hormonal concerns including vaginal discharge, dryness or bleeding.

Blood tests are often normal despite evidence of a local or even distant recurrence and are not recommended as part of regular checkups unless a woman has noticed a new symptom or change in her body. Routine bone or liver scans are not recommended in women without symptoms. Chest x-rays should be done if there are any symptoms that relate to the lungs but not as part of regular follow-up.

The important thing is whether you have symptoms. If you have none, the only regular tests you need are mammograms and regular physical examinations. However, any new or persistent symptom should be investigated.

Mammograms

It is strongly recommended that a set of baseline mammograms be done approximately six months after the completion of treatment.

It is highly unlikely that any cancer recurrence will be detected on this 'baseline' mammogram but by six months, most of the breast changes due to surgery and/or radiation should have settled and a mammogram at that time can serve as a new 'normal' to be used for comparison with future mammograms. Subsequently, mammograms should be done yearly. Not all mammogram abnormalities after treatment are cancer. After radiation and surgery there may be changes in the breast such as scarring or swelling which can be monitored with regular mammograms. Mammograms of the unaffected breast should also be performed once a year.

Ultrasound and MRI

Ultrasounds and MRIs may be helpful if there is something that is not clearly seen on the mammogram but are not recommended as part of the routine follow-up after breast cancer treatment.

For how long should I have regular follow-up visits?

Most recurrences of breast cancer happen in the first two to five years after treatment, but they can occur even 10 to 20 years later. Although five years is not a 'magical' date, we recommend regular visits to a doctor every six months for the first three years after treatment, then every six to 12 months until five years after treatment and then annually as long as you are well. If cancer recurs, the schedule of visits to your doctor will be individualized.

Your responsibilities

You are responsible for some aspects of the follow-up. You may want to learn how to do breast self-examination. This includes examining the uninvolved breast and the radiated breast or the chest wall if a mastectomy has been done. Any new findings or changes should be reported to your doctor. It's important to know that not all changes are due to cancer recurrence. Many women develop thickened areas or redness in a radiated breast, or thickened areas along the scar. Often, it is difficult to know if the thickening is cancerous or not, and a mammogram or biopsy may be necessary. You should show your doctor the area of concern and he or she will do a physical examination and order additional tests if necessary. You should remember to tell any new physicians of your history of breast cancer.

If you notice a new, persisting symptom, make an appointment to see your doctor—don't wait for the next 'routine' appointment several months away. If you are not satisfied that the symptom has been explained, insist on a return visit to your oncologist

CHAPTER THIRTY-EIGHT

Treatment of a local recurrence

A LOCAL OR REGIONAL RECURRENCE refers to a relapse of breast cancer in the breast, the armpit, the skin or muscles of the chest wall or the surrounding lymph nodes. When the cancer recurs in these areas, many patients are surprised and confused. How can the cancer recur after surgery, radiation and chemotherapy? The most likely explanation is that cancer cells present in the skin, muscles or lymphatic system were not removed at the time of mastectomy or partial mastectomy and were not killed by the subsequent treatments.

What are the signs of local or regional recurrences?

Possible signs of local or regional relapse include new lumps, 'thickening' or rashes in the breast, chest wall or armpit or above the collarbone. Recurrence in the lymph nodes in the armpit or behind the collarbone may cause shoulder pain or arm swelling. A new pain that shoots down the arm, or numbness and weakness in the hand or arm may be due to cancer pinching the nerves that extend down into the hand and arm from the neck. Any of these symptoms should prompt an evaluation by a physician.

How are local recurrences treated?

Local relapses often require local treatments such as surgery or radiation, especially if no other recurrence is detected elsewhere in the body. However, if there is evidence that cancer has also recurred elsewhere in the body, the recurrence may be better treated with systemic treatment such as chemotherapy or hormones.

Studies have not been completed to determine whether chemotherapy added to surgery and/or radiation will cure more women with local relapse than surgery and/or radiation alone. Although these trials have not yet shown a definite benefit of adding chemotherapy, if the woman is young and has not had previous chemotherapy, it may be recommended after the local recurrence has been removed.

Cancer recurrence in the breast after partial mastectomy and radiation

Cancer may recur in the breast after conservative surgery and radiation in approximately 2% to 10% of women within 10 years of treatment. Usually, recurrence in the breast can be treated for cure, but this often requires a mastectomy. It is usually not possible to repeat a course of radiation if it was used after the initial surgery. To detect small, curable recurrences, we recommend that a physical examination and mammogram be done every year, starting about six months after completion of the initial surgery, chemotherapy and radiation.

The primary treatment for a small local recurrence is to remove it with surgery if possible. If the local recurrence is too extensive, chemotherapy and hormones are used prior to surgery. Chemotherapy may also be recommended if the woman is young and did not receive chemotherapy at the time of initial diagnosis.

If a local recurrence occurs after partial mastectomy when radiation was not used at the time of initial diagnosis, it can often be treated with a repeat lumpectomy followed by radiation.

Treatment of a local recurrence after mastectomy

Recurrence of breast cancer may occur locally on the chest wall, or regionally in lymph glands in the armpit (axilla), above the collarbone (supraclavicular fossa) or behind the breast bone (internal mammary nodes). If the patient has not previously received radiation, the usual treatment is to remove the recurrence surgically (if it is small and localized) and then give radiation therapy (see Chapter 24). If the recurrence is very extensive, with growth to the bones, muscles or nerves, or cancer recurs within the chest wall and lymph glands after previous radiation therapy, or if recurrence is found at the same time in other organs such as the lungs or bones, treatment needs to be individualized. In these situations it is usual to use hormones or chemotherapy as the first approach.

CHAPTER THIRTY-NINE

Treatment of recurrence elsewhere in the body (metastasis)

Why does the cancer recur elsewhere?

CANCER COMES BACK ELSEWHERE in the body (a 'systemic recurrence') because breast cancer cells escaped into the blood stream prior to the first treatment. Although adjuvant chemotherapy and hormone therapy may have been given to try to destroy these cells, it is not always effective. Cells that are resistant to these treatments are not killed and may divide and grow into detectable cancer metastases.

What can I expect if I have a recurrence elsewhere?

The behavior of the returning cancer depends on a number of factors, including:
- the amount of time passed since the original cancer was diagnosed: a longer time since the diagnosis means the recurrence will grow more slowly,
- the type of initial cancer: the less aggressive, the better
- the tumor's estrogen receptor status: estrogen receptor-positive tumors respond better to treatment than estrogen receptor-negative tumors
- the number of tumor sites: the fewer, the better,

- the sites of the metastases: for example, bone metastases are often slower growing than liver metastases
- the physical state of the woman

The most important factor, however, is how the cancer responds to therapy. If the cancer responds to one type of treatment, then it is more likely that other treatments will also be effective. If the cancer does not shrink in response to any of the usual treatments, the outlook is not as good.

What are the signs of systemic recurrence?

The most common sites for breast cancer to spread are the bones, lungs, liver and brain. Other parts of the body may also be affected including the lymph nodes, skin, eyes, spinal cord, and ovaries. When breast cancer spreads, the cells still look and behave like the original breast cancer. Therefore, if a breast cancer spreads to the lung, it is still breast cancer (not lung cancer). This is important because the types of treatment and the chance of success are different for a spreading breast cancer than, for instance, a lung cancer.

The symptoms of breast cancer metastases depend on the part of the body affected. Cancer in the bones usually causes progressively increasing pain or a spontaneous fracture (a broken bone). In the lungs, it may cause cough or shortness of breath. In the liver it causes loss of appetite, pain in the right upper abdomen and sometimes jaundice. If cancer spreads to the brain it may cause headache, numbness or weakness of an arm or leg, loss of balance, confusion or seizures.

This list of potential problems may be frightening, and a woman may find herself constantly checking for new problems. This is quite normal. Many women report being much more aware of their bodies and of having frequent fears of recurrence, especially in the first year or two after treatment. You should feel comfortable enough to ask your doctors about these concerns. The important things to report are persistent changes. Symptoms that come and go within 24 hours are not a sign of cancer.

What are the goals of treatment of recurrence?

The goals of treatment of metastatic breast cancer are to relieve symptoms, maintain quality of life, and prolong survival. The word 'cure' comes up with hopes for a successful treatment of the systemic recurrence. However, disappointment often follows when the physician cannot guarantee or even predict promising results. Many people live with longstanding (chronic) diseases that cannot be cured, such as heart disease, emphysema, diabetes, and arthritis. Treatment for those conditions is not curative but is given to help avoid severe complications and symptoms. Metastatic breast cancer can be similar to one of these chronic diseases, with a series of treatments given to decrease the symptoms and avoid complications. After a systemic recurrence, breast cancer is usually not curable. However, the length of life can be years and it is impossible to accurately predict how long a particular individual may survive. The average survival after the cancer travels to an organ is about two years but many women live much longer.

The treatments

Patients with metastatic breast cancer usually receive a sequence of treatments, including hormones, radiotherapy, chemotherapy, nutritional support, pain management, psychological support and sometimes surgery.

Systemic (whole body) therapy with hormones or chemotherapy should be given if there are symptoms from the cancer spread or, if the cancer seems to be growing rapidly.

The type of systemic therapy used depends on a number of factors:
- the type of the original tumor: whether it was estrogen or progesterone-receptor-positive and/or HER2 overexpressing
- the length of time since the original diagnosis: even if the initial tumor was estrogen receptor-negative a recurrence occurring many years later may suggest a hormone-responsive cancer
- the organs involved: bone metastases may respond better to hormones
- the severity of the symptoms: if the recurrence is widespread and causing a lot of symptoms then the patient needs the more rapid response that comes with chemotherapy or Herceptin® rather than waiting. Response to hormone therapy may take several months so would not be a good choice in this case.
- the age of the patient: chemotherapy may be too harsh for an elderly woman with other health problems,

• the response to previous therapies: if one hormone therapy had a benefit others may too.

When is hormone therapy used?

For most systemic recurrences the first therapy used is hormones especially if the original breast cancer was estrogen-receptor positive. Even if the original cancer was estrogen receptor-negative, if a few years have passed since that diagnosis, the cancer may respond. The therapies with the fewest side effects are used first, followed by ones that are less well tolerated. Tumors that respond and shrink may stay stable for a long time but at some point recur. If there has been a good response, the initial therapy will be stopped and a new hormone will be tried.

For post-menopausal women, hormonal therapy is usually the first treatment often with an aromatase inhibitor followed by tamoxifen, faslodex or other hormones. (See Chapter 30) Premenopausal women may be treated with tamoxifen, removal of her ovaries or with hormone agents that block the ovarian function.

When is chemotherapy used?

Chemotherapy is used as the first treatment for a systemic recurrence when the tumor is not likely to respond to hormones. This may include a fast-growing tumor, one that occurs soon after the initial diagnosis, or if the original cancer was estrogen receptor-negative. Chemotherapy is also used to treat cancers that have not responded to a trial of hormone therapy or those which initially responded to hormones but are no longer doing so.

For how long is chemotherapy continued?

In recurrent disease, chemotherapy is usually given for two or three cycles and the response is then assessed. If the cancer is responding then treatment may be continued for as long as there is evidence of response and the toxicity is tolerable. If there is not a good response to the first few cycles of chemotherapy, a second type may be tried. If the cancer does not respond to two different types of chemotherapy, it is clearly a very resistant cancer. In this situation the oncologist may decide to avoid further chemotherapy if it is causing side effects and not benefiting the patient.

Often, chemotherapy can effectively decrease the symptoms of metastatic cancer, such as the shortness of breath that may occur if the cancer is in the lungs. It can also reduce symptoms from bone involvement, enlarged lymph nodes, tumors of the skin or liver, or tumors in the abdomen. Unfortunately it can rarely overcome the fatigue that is a common complaint of women with recurrent cancer.

Studies have evaluated high-dose chemotherapy and bone marrow transplants as treatments for women with systemic recurrences. The studies suggest that these strategies are not an improvement over standard-dose chemotherapy, and should not be used except in a research study.

When is radiation used to treat systemic recurrences?

Radiation may be given for recurrent tumors that cause symptoms in a specific area of the body. This includes recurrence in the lymph nodes in the chest that cause shortness of breath, tumors near the esophagus that interfere with swallowing, or tumors in the bones, brain and other structures.

The decision to treat with radiation is based on several factors: the site of the recurrence, the symptoms that may be relieved by the treatment, the symptoms that may be caused by the treatment, and how much radiation, if any, the area has received in the past. Organs in the body tolerate radiation differently. Some areas can only be treated once or can only tolerate low doses of radiation, while other areas can be re-treated or given high doses.

Radiation may be given together with hormones, chemotherapy and/or Herceptin®, or by itself. Radiation is often very successful to decrease pain, particularly bone pain. The relief from pain occurs because radiation kills cancer cells, causing tumors to shrink relieving pressure in the bones. The pain relief may be immediate (a day or two) or gradual (over a month or so). Bones can tolerate high doses of radiation, so if radiation relieved pain once but the pain returns in the same area, the radiation may be repeated with benefit.

The mainstay of treatment for a cancer that recurs in the brain is radiation to the whole brain. The side effects of this therapy include fatigue, mild nausea and headaches which can usually be relieved or prevented with low doses of steroids. Hair loss always occurs when the whole brain is treated with radiation, but it begins to grow back after three or four months.

Occasionally, if a patient has very widespread cancer in the bones and other attempts to gain control have failed, it may be possible to use an agent called strontium. This is a radioactive material, given intravenously that settles in bones and can deliver a whole body dose of radiation. The safety and chance of benefit depends on the health of the bone marrow and the degree of bone activity seen on a bone scan.

Can surgery be used to treat systemic recurrences?

If there are bone metastases, surgery to insert pins or plates may be used to stabilize the bone to avoid fractures, to mend bones that have already broken and to decrease pain. Occasionally, surgery may be used to remove a lump or recurrence on the skin even when there is evidence of other metastases.

If the woman is in reasonable overall shape and has only one site of metastatic disease, surgery can be used to remove it from the lungs, liver or brain, especially in cases of slow-growing tumors. With breast cancer, however, it is rare to have just a single metastasis, so very few patients are considered for this treatment. Since the cancer cells travel in the blood stream, the surgical removal of a single visible lump will not likely cure the cancer because other, smaller clusters of cells that are still too small to be seen, are quite likely to be present elsewhere in the body.

Studies have shown that if there is a solitary metastasis in the brain, doing surgery to remove it if it is easily accessible and then delivering radiation, improves symptom relief and survival compared to radiation alone. The decision to do brain surgery for a woman with metastatic breast cancer needs to be considered carefully. This will involve consultation with a neurosurgeon and radiation oncologist who will consider the tumor's location in the brain and the status of the cancer in the rest of the body.

Another local treatment is chemoablation or radio-frequency ablation of liver metastases. This involves a radiologist inserting a catheter into the liver and injecting medication directly into the tumor or delivering high energy radio waves that heat the tumor to the point of "cooking". Although this technique may shrink the liver tumor, it has some side effects, and does not treat any breast cancer cells outside the liver.

Treatment of fluid accumulation

Recurrent breast cancer can cause excessive fluid to accumulate around the lungs (pleural effusion) due to blockage of normal lymphatic drainage. This can cause shortness of breath or a sharp chest pain that worsens when taking a deep breath. It is usually treated with a 'chest tube' to drain the fluid. Once the fluid is gone, a drug (often doxycycline or bleomycin) or talcum powder is put into the pleural space to close it and prevent the fluid from reaccumulating.

Fluid may also accumulate in the abdomen and cause an uncomfortable swelling of the belly. If the fluid causes discomfort, temporary relief can be obtained if a catheter is inserted into the abdomen to drain the fluid. However, the fluid usually accumulates again very quickly unless some other treatment of the cancer is given, such as chemotherapy or hormone treatment.

What can you do for yourself?

Nutrition

Good nutrition is important to maintain a sense of well-being, but studies have not shown that diet alone can treat metastatic cancer. For many women with a recurrence, eating becomes difficult because they are fatigued or nauseated. In this situation, a registered dietitian may have useful ideas about how to maintain an adequate diet. Chapter 35 discusses some of these issues.

Pain management

Pain may be present during recurrent breast cancer. Radiation and systemic therapy may provide relief but the use of regular and adequate pain medications to avoid letting the pain build up is also important. You will need to find a drug that you tolerate well. With a physician's guidance you can increase the dose until the pain is relieved.

Many patients are uneasy about taking medications for pain, especially narcotics, because they are worried that the pills may be addictive or they feel that taking medication for pain is a sign of 'giving in'. These thoughts are common. Most people will not become addicted to medications that are given to treat pain, and since being pain-free is essential for a good quality of life, it is not a 'weakness' or a sign of 'giving in' to treat the pain. It is simply allowing you to continue as many activities as possible for as long as possible. Unfortunately, all 'pain killers' have side effects. Narcotic medications (codeine, morphine and others) most commonly cause constipation. This can be avoided by taking stool softeners and adequate dietary fiber and fluids as soon as the narcotic medication is started. Bone pain is sometimes decreased by using biphosphonates (clodrinate, pamidronate, etc.).

Mental well-being

Psychological well-being is also an important part of the treatment of recurrent disease. The support of friends and family is crucial, and individual counseling or discussion with a group of women with recurrent cancer may provide a further means of support. Relaxation groups, massage therapy or other types of therapy may also help you cope with this new and frightening situation (see Chapter 36). We encourage women to seek out group support therapy.

Palliative care

Palliative care concentrates on relieving the symptoms caused by the cancer rather than treating the cancer itself. Many centers have specialized palliative care teams that provide in-hospital and home care. These teams work cooperatively with the patient and her family to maintain an optimal quality of life. The goals of palliative care are for the woman to remain comfortably in her own home setting for as long as possible and to enable the woman's independence, dignity and choices during the difficult final phase of her life. Particular attention is paid to pain relief, nutrition, bowel care, psychological support and family needs.

Sadly, the reality is that most women with metastatic breast cancer eventually die of their cancer. Frank discussions between the woman and her family to address her desires regarding her death are important. Decisions such as where she may want to die, funeral arrangements and wills should be made. It is usually better for both the woman and her family to deal with these issues well ahead of the time of need. Knowing that these matters have been settled can sometimes offer a certain peace of mind to all of those involved.

Section Fifteen

Special topics

CHAPTER FORTY

Breast cancer and pregnancy

BREAST CANCER CAN OCCUR DURING PREGNANCY and may be missed as the breasts are engorged and can be difficult to examine.

If breast cancer is diagnosed during pregnancy

If a lump or change appears during pregnancy, the procedure for diagnosing breast cancer is generally the same but extra care is taken to protect the fetus from radiation exposure. Ultrasounds and core biopsies can be done. Mammography can be done with proper shielding of the fetus if necessary. Whole body bone scans should be avoided.

Deciding on a treatment plan

A number of special factors must be considered when treatment of breast cancer during pregnancy, including the stage of the cancer, the type of treatment required, and the gestational age of the fetus. The goal of treatment is to have a good result for both the mother and the baby.

In general, surgical therapy (mastectomy, lumpectomy and axillary dissection) is safe and can proceed. In some circumstances mastectomy is appropriate, with adjuvant treatment delayed until after the birth. Studies have shown that some chemotherapy drugs can be safely given in pregnancy without harming the fetus. The drugs are safer however in the later stages (second and third trimester.) Occasionally, if the cancer is progressing very rapidly, a small risk of harm to the fetus may be accepted and chemotherapy or radiotherapy may be started, even while the fetus is still growing.

An obstetric evaluation should be done to determine the exact age of the fetus and to help decide on the best time for delivery. If the fetus is 32 weeks or older, delivery should be done before the breast cancer treatment starts. A delay in treatment of about four weeks is unlikely to affect the mother's chances of cure, and will allow the baby to mature and have a better chance of being born healthy.

If it is early in the pregnancy, termination may be discussed. Termination does not have an effect on the cancer but may allow earlier treatment with chemotherapy and radiation and in some cases may lessen anxiety for the woman by allowing her to focus on the cancer without fears for her baby.

Some facts about breast cancer and pregnancy

Breast cancer during pregnancy is generally no more aggressive than breast cancer in non-pregnant women of the same age. The survival of women with breast cancer discovered during pregnancy is similar to survival of other women diagnosed at the same age. However, breast cancer in very young women (age <35 years) tends to be more difficult to cure and it can be harder to diagnose during pregnancy so the breast cancer may be more advanced and may therefore have a higher chance of recurrence. Breast cancer does not spread to the fetus. Abortion of the fetus does not improve the outcome or have an effect on the growth of the mother's cancer.

Is fertility affected by breast cancer treatment?

Pre-menopausal women who receive chemotherapy may have their menstrual periods stop permanently and they may become infertile. This is more likely to occur as a woman gets older and nears the time of her normal menopause. Approximately 30% of women under 40 will have a permanent menopause after six months of chemotherapy while for women over 45, permanent menopause is nearly certain after the same treatment. Sometimes menstruation returns six months to a year or more after chemotherapy is completed. Since many women remain fertile while receiving chemotherapy, it is important to use effective methods of contraception (but not birth control pills) if you are sexually active. Radiation, unless it is directed at the pelvis, will not affect fertility. Tamoxifen (hormone therapy) may cause menstrual irregularities but does not make women infertile. It is crucial that women use effective contraception while taking tamoxifen because tamoxifen can harm the fetus.

Even if your menstrual periods are not affected, it is recommended that you do not get pregnant until at least six months after completing treatment, and that you discuss this with your oncologist. Most of the residual effects of chemotherapy and radiation should have resolved by six months.

Pregnancy after breast cancer

Women who get pregnant after having breast cancer have the same long-term cancer outcome as women of the same age who have had breast cancer and do not become pregnant. There is no convincing evidence that getting pregnant makes the cancer re-grow or spread any more frequently or faster than if the woman does not get pregnant. Babies born to women who have had treatment for breast cancer in the past do not have any increased chance of fetal malformations or miscarriages.

Following radiation therapy of the breast, the normal breast tissue is permanently altered. The normal engorgement in preparation for lactation does not occur, and during lactation very little, if any, milk is produced from a radiation-treated breast. This means that the breasts may become quite lopsided during pregnancy as the normal breast enlarges and the radiated breast does not. However, breast-feeding from the unaffected breast is still possible and is encouraged.

Making the decision about whether to become pregnant

Apart from the biological considerations, a woman and her partner need to consider various social, psychological and economic implications of bearing a child. This is doubly hard when the mother-to-be is uncertain of her future. Often, delaying pregnancy for at least six months or more after breast cancer treatment is a good idea. This time gives the woman's body and mind a chance to heal. Some doctors recommend a delay of two to five years to have greater confidence that the cancer won't recur.

CHAPTER FORTY-ONE

Familial breast cancer and genetic testing

Do my daughters have a higher risk of breast cancer?

THIS IS A FREQUENTLY ASKED QUESTION. At the outset, it is important to say that most daughters will not get breast cancer. However, because your daughters are female, this means that they live with at least the 'average' risk of any woman. We also know that breast cancer can be passed on in families (Chapter 3) so the question really becomes, 'How much higher than the normal risk do my daughters face?'

To evaluate your daughter's risk of developing breast cancer several points need to be considered:
- How old were you when you developed breast cancer?
- Did the cancer affect one or both breasts?
- How many of your close relatives have breast cancer?
- How old is your daughter?
- Does your daughter have any other risk factors?

Your age at diagnosis

As women get older, the chance of developing breast cancer increases. This is unrelated to any special inherited tendency (see Chapter 2). Therefore, if the mother develops breast cancer at an older age, for example 75, the daughter's risk is only minimally higher. But if the mother developed cancer in her 30s, it is more likely that something 'genetic' contributed to the cause of the cancer and that her daughter's risk is higher than normal (see Chapter 3).

Cancer of one or both breasts

If both breasts are affected, the chance of a genetic tendency towards breast cancer is higher. If cancer develops in both breasts in a woman younger than 50 years old, it indicates a substantially higher risk (five to 10 times) in her daughters and also in the woman's sisters.

Number of family members with breast cancer

If three or more close blood relatives develop breast cancer, cancer of the ovary or a type of cancer called 'sarcoma', it is more likely that some genetic error is being passed within the family. This increases the risk to the daughter of an affected woman.

Families with a strong history of breast cancer

Approximately 5% to 10% of breast cancers are due to an inherited genetic mutation. Two genes, BRCA1 and BRCA2, have already been identified for breast cancer. The mutations are 'spelling errors' or 'mistakes' on specific chromosomes that have been inherited either from the father or the mother. If a mutation is present, there is a high risk of developing cancer. In these families, relatives in three or more generations are often affected.

Genetic testing can be done to determine if you have inherited a mutation. Once the mutation is identified in someone who has already been diagnosed with breast cancer, the relatives of that person can be tested for that specific mutation. If you are identified as having the altered gene, the lifetime risk of developing breast cancer is 50% to 85% and there is also a higher chance of developing cancer in both breasts. The BRCA1 gene also confers a 45% lifetime risk of ovarian cancer. There is a small increased risk of colon cancer and, for males, prostate cancer. The BRCA2 gene confers an increased risk for both male and female breast cancer as well as ovarian cancer.

These cancers tend to occur five to 10 years earlier in each generation so it is important that planning and screening undertaken early in the lives of women in these families. If an altered gene is identified in family members who have breast cancer, individuals who do not inherit the gene mutation have the same risk for breast cancer as the general population.

Genetic counseling and testing can estimate individual risk

If there is a very strong family history of breast cancer, an unaffected member of the family may be interested in genetic counseling to assess more accurately her individual risk of developing breast cancer. A strong family history is present when there are three or more cases of breast cancer in direct blood relatives, i.e. mother/daughter, aunt/niece, sister, grandmother or a male member of the family. When there is a strong family history of breast cancer on the father's side, it can be passed on to the daughter even though the father does not get cancer himself.

Certain ethnic groups or geographically defined populations have been found to have a high incidence of particular mutations in BRCA1 or BRCA2. For instance, in the general population, one in every 800 individuals might have one of a wide variety of different mutations in BRCA1. In contrast, as many as two in every 100 Ashkenazi Jewish women have been shown to have one of just a few specific mutations. Another example is that a single mutation accounts for most of the cases of inherited breast cancer found in Iceland. These commonly occurring mutations in specific populations are called 'founder mutations.' As more research is done, founder mutations will likely be identified in other ethnic groups or geographic populations.

If you decide to have genetic counseling and testing, you will meet with a medical geneticist and/or genetic counselor who will obtain a detailed family history. Your individual risk for breast cancer can be estimated and you will receive counseling regarding the pros, cons and limitations of genetic testing for the abnormal mutation.

High-risk families: criteria for genetic risk assessment

Genetic testing may identify a mutation in an individual who is:
- a woman with breast cancer diagnosed at age 35 or younger
OR
- a woman with ovarian cancer diagnosed at age 50 or younger
OR
- an Ashkenazi Jewish woman with breast or ovarian cancer diagnosed at any age

252

OR a woman whose family history includes any *two* of the following:

- breast cancer in two or more closely related family members (parents, siblings, children, grandparents, aunts, uncles)
- cancers at an earlier age than expected in the general population (e.g. breast cancer before menopause, prostate cancer before age 50)
- multiple primary cancers in different organs in one individual
- cancers associated with known hereditary syndromes (e.g. breast/ovary,colon/uterus).

Before genetic testing is done, it is important to consider the implications of a positive or negative test, and the decisions you might make with such information. Genetic counseling provides an opportunity to discuss the limitations of genetic testing, how the results might affect you and your family's lives, and how you might use the test results. If you are interested in genetic counseling, have your doctor call your regional cancer center to assess your eligibility and, if appropriate, the best way to make a referral.

Hereditary cancer programs

For women who carry an abnormal mutation for breast cancer such as the BRCA1 or BRCA2 genes, some cancer centers provide a high-risk clinic as part of a Hereditary Cancer Program. In these clinics, women are monitored on a specific surveillance program in which screening and regular physical examinations play an important role in the early detection of cancer. Also, recent studies have shown that some medications may be capable of preventing breast cancer, e.g. tamoxifen (see Chapter 30). Medications may be prescribed for carefully assessed, high-risk individuals.

Screening and Treatment Recommendations

Screening of high risk women with identified or suspected mutations should include an ultrasound of the pelvis every six months to assess the ovaries, and annual mammograms after age 30. Recently MRI scanning has been shown to be effective in women with BRCA1 or BRCA2 mutations. MRIs may pick up earlier changes in young women with dense breasts that cannot be seen well on mammograms.

Periodic breast ultrasound may also be useful. It is recommended that high risk women have a clinical breast examination every six months and mammograms, MRI and breast ultrasounds every 12 months.

Some women at high risk choose to have bilateral mastectomy to decrease their risk of getting a cancer. Prophylactic mastectomy may decrease the risk of developing breast cancer by 98%. Women who have a mastectomy are encouraged to review breast reconstruction options (see Chapter 34).

In some instances, where there is thought to be a genetic influence, removal of the ovaries (oophorectomy) and fallopian tubes may be recommended after a woman has had her children. Oophorectomy decreases the risk of both ovarian cancer and breast cancer. Screening for ovarian cancer with a blood test called CA125, pelvic ultrasounds and pelvic physical examination may not detect ovarian cancer in its early, curable stage.

Prophylactic surgery to decrease cancer risk is an option that needs careful discussion with the oncologist, surgeon and genetic counselor.

CHAPTER FORTY-TWO

Male breast cancer

MEN DEVELOP BREAST CANCER, but it is rare except in families with a BRCA2 gene mutation (see Chapter 41). The cancer usually appears as a lump under the nipple that has been ignored for months or even years. A man with a new breast lump should have bilateral mammograms and a biopsy.

A male's likelihood of surviving breast cancer parallels that of a woman of the same age and stage of disease. Most men (90%) have ER positive cancers. Treatment usually consists of mastectomy and axillary dissection. Radiation may be added if the surgical margins are involved with cancer or if positive lymph nodes are found in the axilla. Tamoxifen, other hormone drugs, and/or chemotherapy are added with the same indications as have been described for a woman of the same age in Chapters 28 and 30. The side effects of treatment for breast cancer in men are much the same as described for women but some hormone drugs may have different side effects related to differences in male hormones. However, men typically present at a later stage than women, so overall, men with breast cancer fare less well than women.

CHAPTER FORTY-THREE

Alternative and complementary treatments

CAUTION: Some complementary or alternative therapies may be useful for cancer patients; however, some may be harmful in certain situations. Intelligent Patient Guide Ltd. urges you to consult with your oncologist before using alternative therapies. Inclusion of an agent, therapy, or resource in this chapter does not imply endorsement by Intelligent Patient Guide Ltd.

What do the terms alternative and complementary mean?

Alternative therapy means treatment that is different from standard therapy. *Complementary therapy* refers to treatment that is designed to supplement standard medical practice.

What are alternative and complementary treatments?

'Alternative' and 'complementary' are terms for a large number of health therapies that are sometimes referred to as 'unproven'. Many of these treatments have value from the point of view of keeping hope alive and giving a woman a sense of control over her life again. But, none of these treatments have been proven to reduce the chance that the cancer will regrow or to shrink cancers that have spread.

Alternative therapy is a catch-all that includes interventions from vitamins to diets, from relaxation and therapeutic touch to herbal remedies, from immune stimulants to metabolic therapy. It is not clear that all these therapies should be lumped into one category, but for the purposes of this chapter, it is useful to discuss their similarities.

It is estimated that over 60% of women with breast cancer use some form of alternative therapy. When vitamins, relaxation methods and visualization are included, the percentage of women using an alternative therapy is probably much larger.

Why are alternative or complementary treatments described as 'unproven'?

Most alternative remedies are referred to as 'unproven' because they have not been subjected to rigorous scientific testing. Physicians depend on extensive experiments and studies to assess new therapies and evaluate their effectiveness. In contrast, the value of alternative therapies is often based on individual testimonials that the therapy was beneficial. This is not very dependable information because the particular circumstances and results cannot be confirmed. Many remedies have not been tested to see if the results can be produced in a consistent way. This is not to say that the treatments have no validity, but most physicians feel uncomfortable placing their faith in a particular remedy without scientific facts to support its use. As well, without more information, it is impossible to know about potential side effects of such treatments—even herbal methods may have severe side effects. It must be acknowledged, however, that much healing occurs outside the realm of science.

Why do patients use non-traditional treatments?

Many women seek alternative therapy when they feel that their physicians predict only 'doom and gloom'. If the oncologist appears to have little to offer or if standard treatments offer only a small chance for cure, it is appealing to try something that seems hopeful and positive. As well, many of the practitioners of holistic approaches are very charismatic and optimistic. Who wouldn't seek the reassurance of a practitioner who gives hope rather than one who seems more negative?

Many women also adopt complementary treatments because they feel empowered in choosing and directing their own care. This is a very positive attitude that helps one's psychological health during the ordeal of cancer therapy. This assertiveness shouldn't be restricted to choosing methods of alternative therapy. Each patient should participate in the decisions regarding her conventional treatment: the type of surgery, radiation, chemotherapy and hormones.

Not only does the patient often feel powerless, but so do many friends and family members, who sometimes steer patients towards alternative treatments because they want to help. Other patients simply have a general mistrust of the conventional medical establishment.

Alternative treatments often seem less toxic and more natural, with claims of boosting the immune system to attack the cancer in a natural way. Many patients claim that holistic programs are gentler, less invasive and more individualized. However, patients must be aware that side effects can still occur.

Types of alternative treatment

The most common alternative cancer therapies can be categorized into the following groups: metabolic therapies, herbal remedies, mega-vitamins, diet therapy, visual imagery and immune therapy. There are also a large number of treatments that cannot be described in detail here, but more complete descriptions are available (see Additional Reading).

Metabolic therapies

The concept of metabolic therapies is that toxins in the body cause and promote cancer, and that certain agents will detoxify the body, including laetrile, iscador (made from mistletoe) and hydrazine. Laetrile was tested in a large study run by the National Cancer Institute in the USA which failed to show that it was beneficial. As well, there have been some laetrile-related deaths, possibly due to the cyanide which is an active ingredient. Studies of hydrazine have not shown a benefit.

Herbal remedies

Herbal remedies have been used by healers for hundreds of years. Some of these remedies have been found to contain active agents that have become modern medicines. These include chemotherapy drugs such as vincristine and vinblastine from the periwinkle plant, paclitaxel from the Pacific Yew tree and acetylsalicylic acid (Aspirin® and others) from the willow tree. Herbal remedies that are promoted for their healing properties include comfrey, taheebo tea and essiac. Essiac, which is now sold under a variety of names such as 'Fluressence®' was used initially by a nurse in Ontario to treat patients with cancer in the 1920s. In the 1980s a company did a scientific study of Essiac, but the results have never been published and are not available. Herbal remedies may not be completely safe; comfrey can cause liver damage and other herbs have been reported to be contaminated by dangerous fungi.

Mega-vitamins

Many people support mega-vitamin use. Vitamins are necessary for many of the chemical reactions in the body. It is claimed that high doses of vitamins, particularly vitamin C, can kill cancer cells and heal tissues. Unfortunately, all vitamins can cause severe side effects if the doses are too high, so a vitamin program should be discussed with your doctor. As well, there have been recent reports of vitamin C interfering with the drugs used in chemotherapy. If you are receiving chemotherapy, very high doses of vitamins should probably be avoided for the days around chemotherapy unless there is proof that there is no interaction between the vitamins and chemotherapy. Two studies have shown that patients with lung cancer who received high-dose beta-carotene had more cancer recurrences than patients not receiving beta-carotene. This suggests that high-dose beta-carotene may in fact be harmful. There is no evidence that the vitamin doses in a multi-vitamin tablet are harmful.

Diet

'You are what you eat' is a phrase we have all heard. With respect to cancer, diet has been suggested as a cause by some and as a treatment by others. Various diets have been proposed as therapies for cancer. These include macrobiotic diets, vegetarian diets, grape diets, the Mormon diet and many others. However, without there being a simple cause for cancer, it is difficult to imagine that a diet alone can cure all malignancies; on the other hand, dietary changes may be helpful in promoting overall health (see Chapter 35). There is one recent study however suggesting that a low fat diet may decrease the risk of breast cancer recurrence.

Immune therapy

Many treatments can be included in this group. These all depend on the theory that cancer is due to an immune defect, so if the immune system can be strengthened, then the cancer can be controlled. Although some cancers do seem to be directly related to the immune system, others occur without any obvious connection to our immune system, which is a very complex and poorly understood part of our make-up. Researchers and immunologists are struggling to determine what role the immune system has in the treatment of various cancers. At this time, despite years of research, there are many unanswered questions. Vaccines and medications to boost the immune system have validity for some cancers, but there is no evidence at this time that immune stimulation is beneficial against breast cancer.

Visual imagery and other forms of 'mental energy'

The concept of visual imagery is that mental energy can be focused through visualization to destroy cancer cells or stop their growth. Relaxation groups and meditation rely on the premise that a healthy mental attitude can aid healing. As well, other methods such as therapeutic touch, massage therapy and other physical techniques rely on the concept of the connection between mental attitude and physical health. While these therapies have not been proven to act on their own, they promote one's sense of responsibility and control in a way that can act with other healing remedies. The field of neuroendocrinology explores the connection between stress, health and the immune system and may lead to some important discoveries and treatments.

What are the risks of these treatments?

The risks of alternative therapies are related to the lack of scientific testing. We depend on regulations to keep our food safe. We test and categorize which additives are approved, and legally require that they be listed on the box or package to protect us as consumers. None of these safeguards exist for alternative cancer treatments. As well, the costs can be prohibitive. A therapy that promises a 'cure' makes people with cancer susceptible to paying potentially large amounts of money for something with no firm evidence of benefit.

The practitioners of alternative treatments may be very ethical and well-meaning, but there are no safeguards to protect patients from quacks and crooks that are also in the business.

Another problem is that if the cancer does not respond to a change in, say, behavior or diet, the patient may feel like a failure. Many people already (mistakenly) feel completely responsible for getting cancer in the first place—due to their diet, or stress in their past. Although accepting responsibility for making treatment choices is worthwhile, blaming oneself can be very damaging.

Finally, some cancers are very treatable and can be cured with standard therapy. Although every patient should have a choice of treatment, there are concerns that when curative treatment is rejected in favor of an alternative therapy, the chance of being cured may be lost because of a delay in initiating anti-cancer treatment of proven benefit.

Ongoing studies of complementary therapy on its own and in combination with conventional treatments may provide the information necessary to properly assess and recommend various treatments. We eagerly await the results.

Open discussion builds trust

Many patients are hesitant to discuss their interest in alternative methods of cancer treatment with their doctors. However, it is important that the physician be informed for the benefit of both the patient and the doctor.

Patients who opt for alternative or complementary treatments should not be hesitant to maintain contact and receive treatment from their conventional doctors or to return to them when the time seems right.

CHAPTER FORTY-FOUR

Clinical research: Looking for better answers

Why are clinical studies important?

AS MOST WOMEN QUICKLY LEARN, there are a lot of unanswered questions about breast cancer. What is/are the cause(s)? Can we prevent it? What new treatment or approach might give better results than we're getting right now? Is there some way of curing breast cancer permanently?

Research studies (also called 'trials') try to answer these and other questions. It's an ongoing process, with questions constantly being asked, and researchers continually looking for better ways of treating patients. Sometimes we forget that the treatments we now consider as "standard" for breast cancer (drugs, surgery, radiation) were at one time considered experimental. It is because women with breast cancer have volunteered to participate in research studies that the current treatments are available.

What are the steps in testing a new treatment?

All potential treatments go through the same type of rigorous evaluation process that can be illustrated with the example of the testing of a new drug.

All new drug treatments begin in the laboratory. If extensive tests in test tubes and mice show that a new drug has potential in treating breast cancer, then it is tested in humans in a preliminary (phase 1) study to check side effects and to establish a dose level at which side effects are acceptable. The drug is then tested in a small group of women to determine its effect in controlling the cancer (phase 2). In this phase the question is, 'Does the drug work at a dose that is safe in humans?' Phase 1 and 2 studies usually involve volunteers with advanced or metastatic breast cancer.

If the results are still promising, the question then arises whether the new drug is better than the 'standard' treatment. To determine this, a third (phase 3) study is done in which women are randomly selected for either the new or old treatment. If it is not known which treatment is superior, it is ethical to compare the treatments in consenting, volunteer women with breast cancer.

Scientific studies such as these must follow rigid statistical rules to confirm that the information gained is reliable and valid. It is also important to know that patients must give their consent before they are included in any study.

Other treatments can be tested in a similar fashion. For example, ongoing studies are evaluating radiation of the lymph nodes, the appropriate role of sentinel lymph node biopsy, the optimum period of time for giving hormonal therapy and the role of exercise to improve quality of life and tolerance to treatment during chemotherapy.

Media reports about advances in understanding cancer or new treatments are often based on very preliminary data. Sometimes, a promising phase 2 study or even an animal study may be reported as a 'clinical' breakthrough. This is confusing for the public and physicians as well. Until a new treatment can be confirmed to be both effective and superior to standard therapy in large studies, it cannot be recommended as the new standard of care. However, with persistence and with the participation of patient volunteers, new therapies are being introduced every year.

What should I do if I'm asked to be part of a study?

Participation in any study is voluntary. If you are asked to consider enrolling in a study, you should understand why the study is being done, what is already known of the treatment's side effects and benefits, and what the alternatives are. Many phase 2 and 3 trials use treatments that have been available for some time, so there could be considerable information available. On the other hand, it is important to understand that the primary aim of a phase 1 trial is to define the side effects of a novel treatment, since usually very few patients have received this treatment.

Before any study is done, hospital ethics committees evaluate the research plan to ensure that the rights of the patient are protected and that the study is ethical in its design and implementation. These ethics committees always include members of the lay public. Informed consent must be obtained from each patient before enrolment in the study. This means that the researcher must carefully discuss the study with each potential participant, explaining the reasons for it, the risks and benefits, and other options the patient has in terms of treatment. The patient should not sign consent to participate unless she has had all her questions answered thoroughly.

Ultimately, each woman is free to decide what is in her best interest, and must be comfortable in choosing whether to take part in a study. Also, she must understand that her standard of care will not change if she subsequently decides to withdraw from it. It is through the commitment of thousands of women participating in clinical research that many advances have been made in the treatment of breast cancer.

CHAPTER FORTY-FIVE

Awareness and advocacy

THE GOOD NEWS IS that most of us live after an encounter with breast cancer. The tough news is that we still can't expect everyone to be cured and we can't reassure our daughters that breast cancer is preventable. When I was in high school, my friend Cathy's mum developed breast cancer and had radical surgery. Thankfully, surgical techniques have improved, and today the type of surgery she endured has almost totally disappeared. We knew that one side of her body was disfigured, that the arm on her affected side was swollen and painful, and that she was very, very sick. We whispered about 'it' behind Cathy's back, but never asked her how everything was at home. We weren't heartless, only young, frightened, embarrassed and unable to find the right words. In retrospect, I realize that we figured that if we denied that the life of one of our favorite mums was being threatened, that breast cancer would go away and leave us, and our own mums, unscathed.

Decades later, with close to one and a half decades of survival under my belt, I know that silence and denial kill. Our job as advocates has been to break the silence and focus an uncompromising light on all the issues surrounding breast cancer.

The physical and emotional effects of this disease can be devastating. While each of us experiences breast cancer differently, most of us ride a roller coaster of overwhelming anxiety, grief, sadness, anger, frustration, hope, denial, black humor...and the fear of a truncated future.

On our bodies, there's an indelible physical reminder that our lives have been put in peril, and that breast cancer may return to threaten our lives once again, and perhaps kill us. Advocacy offers a means to channel our energies and to do something positive about a situation over which we still have no means of prevention and precious little control. It's a way to save lives and to forge purpose out of an apparently chaotic, senseless situation.

Most of us who develop breast cancer are taken by surprise, with no family history or obvious risk factors. We face an instant medical crash course in learning enough about the disease to make critical treatment choices. Usually, it's not until the immediate crises of diagnosis and treatment decisions have passed that an awareness of the staggering scope of breast cancer becomes apparent. When the huge number of women affected become apparent, a "Why me?" cry turns into a "why not me?" realization.

With breast cancer we confront the uncomfortable issue of breasts and the values of femininity, sexuality and nurturing we have placed upon them. We relish memories of babies nursing at our breasts, lovers' caresses and holding those we cherish in a soft embrace. On every newsstand, in every movie and TV show, we are swamped with images exploiting cleavage, with never-ending expectations of how a woman must look to be womanly. It is essential to get rid of any embarrassment you might have over having breast cancer. The public needs to know that treating breast cancer is about saving life, and that even with changed bodies, life, love, sex and femininity carry on. Indeed, a re-evaluation of priorities and values in the shadow of breast cancer may yield a more conscious appreciation of life. Believe me, no one signs on for cancer to have a 'growth experience,' but it often happens.

Advocacy comes in many forms. We need to corner the politicians who control health care and research purse strings to determine how much money has been targeted for breast cancer and how it is being spent. Charitable organizations should be questioned on their spending priorities. We need to know how recent research has benefitted patients in screening centers, clinics and hospitals.

Breast cancer has been around for centuries and has received a great deal of attention over the past decade. So, why does it remain a hot, public topic? Is it because our rapidly aging population, with active, educated and influential women, is edging into the most susceptible age brackets? Is it because sexual issues are more in the open? Is it because of the continuing public awareness that more money is still needed for breast cancer research, education and swift treatment? Is it due to the pointed questions about why there hasn't been more progress in finding preventive strategies and cures, even though the media tout cancer cure 'breakthroughs' on a regular basis?

It is also our job to inform women of the realities of breast cancer and to encourage them to take realistic care of themselves. It is true that thousands of Canadian women have had their futures stolen from them and die prematurely every year of the disease. It is also true that over 2,000,000 North American women are living with a previous diagnosis of breast cancer and are hoping that it never returns.

It is tragic that too many women in their most vulnerable years, 50 and over, are not yet using the mammographic programs available to them. The age for beginning screening is no longer controversial. Although it's not yet the 100% perfect, early detection system, I am grateful, as are so many other women, that my tumor was found in my mid 40's, earlier than it would otherwise have been without this technology. Without it, my tumor would have remained an undetected time bomb in my body for months or years, and I would likely have been faced with much more difficult treatment.

Across North America, information is not easily available in the languages of smaller cultural groups. Not all women know how to perform breast self-examination. Not all women know that, if they are diagnosed, there are treatment options and that the earlier the diagnosis, the better the options will be. Not all women realize that their doctors are there to serve them and that they have rights to full information, their own personal medical records, second opinions and choices. Not all families know that genetic screening clinics are available to give excellent information on the potential susceptibility of women whose families included generations of women who were previously affected by the disease. Our moral support and willingness to accompany others through the maze of new, complex information and difficult choices is a front-line form of advocacy.

The most basic tools of advocacy are information, facts, figures and a clear understanding of the social and financial impact of the disease. However, breast cancer cannot be 'sold' on finances and statistics alone. The personal is political, and stories of women and families facing breast cancer must be told. The pain of lost battles must be made real and the hope that comes from the lives of long-time survivors spread. As advocates, we must recognize that influence is created and decisions are based on gut reactions as well as logic.

So, what can only one person do?

- Educate yourself before you do anything. Learn as much as you can about the disease and the issues that interest you. For example, if funding is your concern, find out how funds are being spent by reading annual general reports of groups raising money. Find out how much money is being spent on administration and how much is going directly to further the cause. Apply to be part of grant-allocation committees. Ask for a 'report card' on previous grants. What has been learned? Or, as another example, if long waiting lists are your issue, ensure you get the correct, current statistics. Incorrect information will weaken your effectiveness.

- Focus. Advocacy comes in many forms: support groups, fund raising, education, raising concerns about genetic testing, political lobbying and ensuring mammography clinics have the best equipment. Keep your goals clear. Be bold in asking people with the skills you need to help you.

- Find others. Place an ad in the local newspaper asking for others interested in the cause to contact you. Host a meeting. Many an influential group has first started around a kitchen table. Create a website and link to other groups. Buddies help. As one of the founding paddlers of *Abreast in a Boat*, the first internationally competitive dragon boat team entirely powered by breast cancer survivors, I know that personal support and public advocacy are close kin. One can power the other. What started out in Canada with 24 women paddlers in one experimental boat has morphed into over 90 crews world wide, from Canada to Poland, from Singapore to New Zealand. These teams won't be ignored and the numbers of boats are dwarfed by the thousands of aware supporters cheering their efforts and becoming educated about the numbers of people affected by the disease.

- Network strategically. Consider joining your group with other breast cancer groups locally, provincially, nationally and internationally. Consider cross-marketing and co-operative events. Through the web, learn from the success of other advocacy organizations whether concerned with breast cancer or other issues. Join a virtual group.
- Make friends with the media and make it easy for the media to follow your progress. Look for 'photo opportunities' and take pictures of events. Write brief 'personal interest' stories. Cultivate specific TV, radio and print contacts and educate them on your cause with concise, factual information sheets. Find a credible spokesperson.
- Speak out courageously in public, especially at election time. This is the time to hold their feet to the fire. Ask each political party the same, specific, tough questions you want answered. Compare their answers. For example, how would each party deal with long hospital and surgical waiting lists? Will they fund new drug therapies?

The job of finding the cause(s) and ways to prevent breast cancer is a team effort, resembling a marathon more than a sprint. Our researchers, nurses, clinicians, and everyone else on our medical teams are people with families and financial obligations like the rest of us. Their skills are being sought internationally. Like it or not, we have to compete for their expertise. We need to continue to attract sustained, secure funding and to convince our governments and charitable organizations to set priorities. What could be more important than putting corporate donations and tax dollars to work to save bodies and lives?

Even if we had a magic bullet, a magic cure for all forms of breast cancer right now, we would still have to treat women currently diagnosed and we would have to scour the country to find others who have the disease hidden in their bodies. So, we need a prevention strategy. Our job in all this will require determined optimism.

APPENDIX

Breast self-examination technique

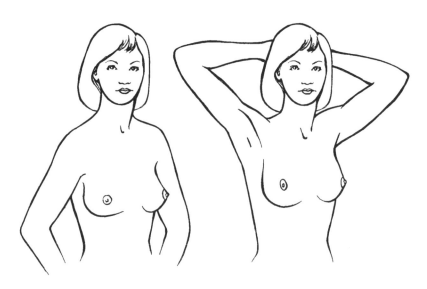

Standing, arms down, to
check basic appearance.

Raising arms to
look for changes.

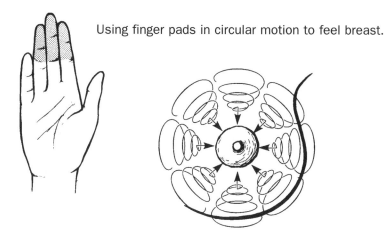

Using finger pads in circular motion to feel breast.

Lying flat on the back and feeling breast again.

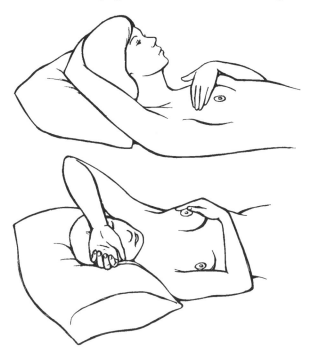

Lying slightly to each side to feel breast.

Glossary

Adjuvant therapy: Treatment that is given in addition to the initial, apparently complete surgery to help prevent the cancer from recurring. Often called 'insurance' against recurrence of cancer. Adjuvant therapy is given after surgery, whereas neoadjuvant therapy is given prior to surgery (see neoadjuvant therapy).

Androgen: Male hormone that may be used as a drug to treat breast cancer.

Angiogenesis: Literally "new blood vessel growth" from the Greek 'angio' = "vessel" and 'genesis' = "birth or growth". Angiogenesis is a required part of cancer growth because the new blood vessels are necessary to bring a supply of oxygen and nutrients to the cancer cells.

Aromatase: An enzyme located in the fat and other body tissues that is involved in the production of estrogen from other steroid hormones, in postmenopausal women.

Aromatase Inhibitors: Drugs that can block the action of the aromatase enzyme. This block decreases the production of estrogen in postmenopausal women. These drugs are used as 'hormone' treatments in postmenopausal women with tumors that are estrogen receptor positive. Common aromatase inhibitors are anastrozole (Arimidex®), letrozole (Femara®), and exemestane (Aromasin®).

Atypical cells: Cells that appear abnormal but not frankly cancerous when viewed under the microscope.

Axilla: The underarm area between the armpit and the collarbone.

Benign tumor: A harmless tumor that is not cancerous.

Biopsy: A procedure in which a small piece of tissue is removed to be studied under the microscope to help make a diagnosis. A biopsy may be done using surgery (an open biopsy) or with a fine or core needle inserted in the doctor's office or using ultrasound or mammographic guidance.

Brachytherapy: The use of catheters or radio-active pellets directly inserted into the breast to deliver radiation internally to the tissue surrounding the tumor or surgical cavity.

Breast implant: A round or tear drop-shaped sac filled with salt water or silicone that is placed under the skin and muscle of the chest wall after mastectomy to create a breast shape or improve the shape of an existing breast.

Breast prosthesis: An artificial breast form that can be worn externally to replace the breast shape after a mastectomy.

Breast reconstruction: Surgical procedures (several types) that create a breast shape with or without a nipple after breast surgery for cancer. This may involve insertion of a breast implant or creation of a breast shape from other body tissues.

Calcifications: Tiny deposits of calcium that may signify cancer and can be seen on a mammogram.

Carcinoma: Another word for cancer.

Cancer: The abnormal and uncontrolled growth of cells that may invade and destroy surrounding tissues.

Chemotherapy: Treatment for cancer involving the use of drugs

Circulating cells: Free floating cancer cells found in a blood sample.

Clinical trial: A research study designed to test a new therapy or treatment approach.

Cyst: A non-cancerous sac or lump filled with fluid.

Dissection: Surgical cutting open of a part of the body.

Duct ectasia: Widened (or dilated) milk ducts.

Edema: Swelling of body tissue due to accumulation of fluid. This may occur in the arm or breast after removal of lymph nodes during treatment for breast cancer.

Estrogen: A sex hormone that is responsible for the development of female characteristics such as breasts and broadening of the hips at the time of puberty. Estrogen has a key role in the menstrual cycle and pregnancy and stimulates the growth of some breast cancers. It is made in the ovaries before menopause and to a lesser extent, throughout the body fat after menopause.

Estrogen receptor (ER): A protein in the cancer cell that binds to the hormone estrogen. A cancer cell that is estrogen receptor-rich (or positive) is usually sensitive to hormones.

Fat necrosis: A lump of dead fat cells in the breast that is often tender and may occur after an injury severe enough to cause bruising such as a car accident, physical abuse or breast surgery

Fibroadenoma: A firm, round, fibrous lump, most often found in young women and which does not turn cancerous.

Fine needle aspiration biopsy: A biopsy technique in which a thin needle is inserted into the body and a few cells or some fluid is removed for diagnosis.

Fine wire localization: A technique to direct a surgical biopsy to an area of the breast which is abnormal on a mammogram but which cannot be felt. A thin wire is placed into the breast under ultrasound or mammographic control to guide the surgeon to the correct part of the breast

HER2: A cancer gene (oncogene) that is overexpressed (makes too much HER2 protein). Found in approximately 20% of breast cancers. This oncogene may cause the cancer to be more aggressive. Also called the Her2/neu gene.

Herceptin®: An anti-HER2 antibody that is useful in controlling some breast cancers that overexpress HER2 (see HER2).

Hormone therapy: Treatment for breast cancer that involves altering the hormone levels in the body. This may involve removing the ovaries or the use of specific drugs given as tablets or injections.

Hormones: Normally occurring chemicals produced by specific parts of the body (glands) that travel through the blood stream to another location in the body where they cause a change in a structure or function of a body tissue (e.g. estrogen in young women is produced in the ovaries and causes the breasts to develop).

Hyperplasia: Cells that divide and accumulate in excessive numbers but are not yet cancerous.

In situ breast cancer: Cancer growing within the milk ducts or milk glands of the breast.

Invasive cancer: Cancer that has extended or spread out of the milk ducts to invade adjacent tissues or organs.

Lobules (lobular): That part of the breast housing the milk glands.

Lumpectomy: A surgical procedure in which the tumor and a small margin of surrounding normal breast tissue is removed. Lumpectomy may also be called a partial mastectomy, segmental mastectomy, wide excision or breast conserving surgery.

Lymph nodes: Small lima bean-shaped structures grouped at various locations along the lymph system in the body (e.g. armpits, neck, groin). They act as the main 'filters' to defend against infections and can be a site for cancer to spread. Lymph nodes under the arm are frequently removed as part of breast cancer surgery to determine if cancer has spread beyond the breast.

Lymphatic system: The network of vessels throughout the body that carries lymph fluid to and from all the tissues of the body.

Lymphedema: See Edema.

Magnetic Resonance Imaging (MRI): A body scan using strong magnetic fields to examine internal body structures.

Malignant tumor: A cancerous lump that is harmful because it grows out of control and invades and destroys surrounding tissues and can spread to other parts of the body (metastasize).

Mammogram: An x-ray of the breast.

Mastectomy: A surgical procedure in which the whole breast is removed. May be a modified radical, radical, simple or subcutaneous mastectomy. For partial mastectomy see Lumpectomy.

Menopause: The time of life when a woman's monthly periods stop because her ovaries have stopped making estrogen.

Metastases: The spread of a cancer from one organ where growth started, to another part of the body. (also as a verb—to metastasize)

Microcalcifications: Very tiny calcifications.

Mutation: An alteration in a gene which causes the gene to function abnormally.

Neoadjuvant therapy: Radiation, chemotherapy or hormonal therapy given prior to surgery to enhance the effect of surgery or to make the surgery easier. Neoadjuvant therapy is given prior to surgery, whereas adjuvant therapy is given after surgery.

Necrosis: The death of cells.

Oncologist: A doctor who specializes in the treatment of patients with cancer.

Palpation: Examination with the hands; to feel.

Papillomas: Small growths inside the milk duct that are benign, but may cause bleeding from the nipple.

Partial breast radiation: A technique to deliver radiation to just the quarter of the breast thought to be most at risk of cancer recurrence.

Pathologist: A doctor who specializes in the diagnosis of disease by studying the structure and function of normal and abnormal cells and tissues of the body.

Predictive factor: A test or cancer characteristic (e.g. Estrogen receptor or HER2 status) that predicts the likelihood that a cancer will respond to a particular treatment (e.g. Estrogen receptor status predicts response to hormone therapy; HER2 status predicts response to the drug Herceptin®).

Primary cancer: A cancer in the organ of origin.

Progesterone: A female sex hormone involved in a number of functions, including the menstrual cycle and pregnancy.

Progesterone receptor (PR): A protein in the cancer cell that, together with the ER status, indicates the likelihood that a breast cancer will respond to a hormone.

Prognosis: An estimate of the expected course of the disease.

Prognostic factor: A test or cancer characteristic (e.g. size of the tumor, grade or number of lymph nodes involved) that indicates the likelihood of future cancer re-growth.

Prophylactic: A preventive treatment which may involve any type of therapy, e.g. drugs, surgery, radiation.

Prosthesis: An artificial device that is attached to the body to substitute for a part of the body that is missing.

Radiotherapy (radiation therapy, RT): The use of high-energy radiation for the treatment of cancer.

Recurrence: The reappearance or regrowth of cancer. The recurrence may be in the original site (a local recurrence), in the adjacent lymph nodes (a regional recurrence) or elsewhere in the body (a systemic or distant recurrence).

Remission: When there is no detectable evidence of cancer on physical examination or with medical tests.

Risk factor: Something that increases the chance of getting a disease. A risk factor may be either acquired from the environment or inherited.

Sarcoma: A type of cancer arising from the connecting tissues of the body (e.g. the muscles, bones, nerves, fatty tissues).

Sclerosing adenosis: Scarring and inflammation around the breast glands that may show up as fine calcifications on a mammogram.

Screening: Tests done on a well person to detect unsuspected disease.

Secondary cancer: A cancer that has spread to another site. Also called 'metastatic cancer.'

Sentinel node: The lymph node closest to or receiving the first lymph drainage from the breast, usually in the axilla (armpit).

Sentinel node biopsy: A technique to identify the lymph node most likely to be involved if cancer has spread outside the breast. It involves injecting blue dye and/or a radio-active tracer around the tumor and tracing the lymph flow to the nearest (or sentinel) lymph node.

Staging: The clinical examinations and tests done at the time of diagnosis to determine the extent of the cancer in the body.

Subcutaneous: The area immediately below the skin.

Sutures: Stitches used to close up a surgical wound.

Systemic: Affecting the body in general rather than one specific part.

Tamoxifen: An anti-estrogen drug and the most widely used 'hormone therapy' to treat breast cancer metastases and/or help prevent the recurrence of breast cancer.

Tumor: Any abnormal growth of tissue. Can be cancerous (malignant) or non-cancerous (benign).

White blood cells: Cells in the blood stream that detect and fight infection, 'foreign' material and abnormal cells.

Additional Reading

Body image / breast reconstruction

100 questions and answers about breast surgery. / Disa, Joseph J;
Keuchel, Marie Czenko. Sudbury, MA: Jones and Bartlett Publishers,
2006.

*Breast reconstruction guidebook : issues and answers from research to
recovery.* / Steligo, Kathy. San Carlos, CA: Carlo Press, 2003.

Breast reconstruction using the TRAM flap (videocassette or DVD). /
Bowman, Cameron. Vancouver, BC: Banford Communications, 2003.

*Classical stretch : the Esmonde technique : breast cancer : rehabilitation
post-surgery* (videocassette or DVD). / Esmonde-White, Miranda.
Montreal, QC: Classical Stretch, 2002.

*Show me : a photo collection of breast cancer survivors' lumpectomies,
mastectomies, breast reconstructions and thoughts on body image*
2nd ed. / Milton S. Hershey Medical Center, Pennsylvania State
University. Hershey, PA: Milton S. Hershey Medical Center, 2001.

Complementary and alternative therapy

National Center for Complementary and Alternative Medicine website.
http://nccam.nih.gov/

*Breast cancer: beyond convention : the world's foremost authorities on
complementary and alternative medicine offer advice on healing.* /
Debu Tripathy and Isaac Cohen. New York NY: Atria Books, 2003.

*American Cancer Society's guide to complementary and alternative
cancer methods* / American Cancer Society. Atlanta, GA: American
Cancer Society, 2000.

*Complementary cancer therapies : combining traditional and alterna-
tive approaches for the best possible outcome* / Labriola, Dan.
Roseville, CA: Prima Health, 2000.

Unconventional cancer therapies manual (online version). Vancouver,
BC: BC Cancer Agency, 2000.
http://www.bccancer.bc.ca/PPI/UnconventionalTherapies/default.htm

Complementary therapies : empowering the cancer patient (videocassette). / Donnelly, Laurie. Woburn, MA: Xenejenex Productions, 1998.

Coping / relaxation / support

Picking up the pieces : moving forward after cancer. / Magee, Sherri; Scalzo, Kathy - Vancouver, BC: Raincoast Books, 2006.
Anatomy of hope : how people prevail in the face of illness. / Groopman, Jerome E. New York, NY: Random House, 2004.
You are never alone : prayers and meditations to sustain you through breast cancer. / Murray, Maureen. Pittsburgh, PA: Oncology Nursing Society, 2004.
After breast cancer : a common-sense guide to life after treatment. / Schnipper, Hester Hill; Schnipper, Lowell E. New York: Bantam Books, 2003.
After breast cancer : answers to the questions you're afraid to ask. / Mayer, Musa. Sebastopol, CA: O'Reilly & Associates, Inc. 2003.
Helping your mate face breast cancer: tips for becoming an effective support partner for the one you love during the breast cancer experience. 5th ed. / Kneece, Judy C. West Columbia, SC: EduCare Inc. 2003.
Living beyond breast cancer : a survivor's guide for when the treatment ends and the rest of your life begins. / Weiss, Marisa C; Weiss, Ellen. New York, NY: Times Books, 1998.

Fitness / exercise / lymphedema

Lymphedema : understanding and managing lymphedema after cancer treatment. / American Cancer Society. Atlanta, GA: American Cancer Society, 2006.
Breast cancer survivor's guide to fitness (DVD). / Kaelin, Carloyn; Gardiner, Josie; Prouty, Joy. Boston, MA: Brigham and Women's Hospital, 2005.
Lymphedema : a breast cancer patient's guide to prevention and healing. 2nd ed. / Burt, Jeannie; White, Gwen. Alameda, CA: Hunter House Inc., Publishers, 2005.
Thriving after breast cancer : essential healing exercises for body and mind. / Davis, Sherry Lebed; Gunning, Stephanie. New York, NY: Broadway Books, 2002.
Essential exercises for breast cancer survivors. / Halverstadt, Amy; Leonard, Andrea. Boston, MA: Harvard Common Press, 2000.

General information

Dr. Susan Love's breast book. 4th ed. / Love, Susan; Lindsey, Karen. Cambridge, MA: Da Capo Press, 2005.

Mayo Clinic guide to women's cancers / Hartmann, Lynn C; Loprinzi, Charles L. Rochester, MN.: Mayo Clinic, 2005.

100 questions and answers about breast cancer / Brown, Zora; Leffall, LaSalle D; Platt, Elizabeth. Boston, MA: Jones and Bartlett Publishers, 2003.

Breast cancer sourcebook : basic consumer health information about breast cancer, including diagnostic methods, treatment options, alternative therapies, self-help information, statistical and demographic data and facts for men with breast cancer : along with reports on current research initiatives, a glossary of related medical terms, and a directory of sources for further help and information / Prucha, Edward J; Bellenir, Karen. Holmes, PA: Omnigraphics, Inc. 2001.

Healthy eating

Staying alive! : cookbook for cancer free living : real survivors— real recipes— real results. / Errey, Sally and Simpson, Trevor. Vancouver, BC: Bellisimo Books, 2003.

Dietitian's cancer story : information and inspiration for recovery and healing from a 3-time cancer survivor. 8th ed. / Dyer, Diana. Ann Arbor, MI: Swan Press, 2002.

What to eat when you don't feel like eating. Haller, James. Hantsport, NS: Lancelot Press Limited, 2002.

Nutrition during and after cancer treatment : a guide for informed choices by cancer survivors. American Cancer Society Workgroup on Nutrition and Physical Activity for Cancer Survivors. *CA Cancer J Clin 2001;51:153-181.* Available online: http://www.cancer.org/docroot/pub/content/pub_3_8x_nutrition_during_and_after_cancer_treatment.asp

Nutrition and breast cancer: What you need to know (booklet). Canadian Cancer Society, 2004. Available online: http://www.cancer.ca/ccs/internet/publicationlist/0,,3172_247810668_271268337_langId-en.html

The cancer survival cookbook: 200 quick & easy recipes with helpful eating hints. 2nd. ed. / Donna L. Weihofen and Christina Marino. Toronto, ON: John Wiley & Sons, Inc. 2002

American Cancer Society's healthy eating cookbook : a celebration of food friends and healthy living. 2nd. ed. Atlanta, GA: American Cancer Society, 2001.

Personal stories

Run your own race : Dr. Marla's journey with breast cancer (DVD). / Shapiro, Marla; 90th Parallel Film and Television Productions Ltd. Toronto, ON: CTV News, 2005.

Fighting for our future : how young women find strength, hope, and courage while taking control of breast cancer. / Murphy, Beth. New York, NY: McGraw-Hill, 2003.

How to ride a dragon : women with breast cancer tell their stories. / Tocher, Michelle. Toronto, ON: Key Porter Books, 2002.

It takes a worried man : a memoir. / Halpin, Brendan. New York, NY: Villard Books, 2002.

Ice bound : a doctor's incredible battle for survival at the south pole. / Nielsen, Jerri. New York, NY: Hyperion, 2001

Uplift : secrets from the sisterhood of breast cancer survivors. / Delinsky, Barbara. New York, NY: Washington Square Press, 2001.

Survivor's guide to breast cancer. / Chang, Alice F.; Spruill, Karen Mang. Oakland, CA: New Harbinger Publications, Inc. 2000.

Before I say goodbye. / Picardie, Ruth; Seaton, Matt; Picardie, Justine. Toronto, ON: Penguin Books, 1998.

Sexuality

Sexuality and cancer : for the woman who has cancer, and her partner / Schover, Leslie R. New York, NY: American Cancer Society, Inc. 2001. Online version revised 2004: http://documents.cancer.org/6710.00/

More detailed medical information

Breast cancer. 2nd ed. (textbook) / Winchester, David J. Hamilton, ON: B.C. Decker Inc. 2006.

Diseases of the breast. 3rd ed. (textbook) / Harris, Jay R. Philadelphia, PA: Lippincott Williams & Wilkins, 2004.

Clinical practice guidelines for the care and treatment of breast cancer : a Canadian consensus document developed by the Steering Committee on Clinical Practice Guidelines for the Care and Treatment of Breast Cancer (online resource including updates). Ottawa, ON : Canadian Medical Association, 2004. http://www.cmaj.ca/cgi/content/full/158/3/DC1

Index

Tumor. *See also* Biopsy; Neoadjuvant
therapy; Pathology report
classification, 71–73
description in pathology report, 65
hormone receptors, 72, 163–164
markers, in blood tests, 82
size, 73
staging, 81–84
surgical issues, 101–102
Tylenol, 152

U

Ultrasound
cancer screening, during pregnancy,
247
core biopsy, 56
"core needle" biopsy of cysts, 47, 48
fine needle aspiration biopsy, 51–52,
56
for high-risk women, with familial
breast cancer gene, 253, 254
not recommended as follow-up after
treatment, 231
purpose, 47
screening for breast cancer, 34, 47–48

V

Vagina
bleeding, 173, 175, 176
discharge, as side effect of treatment,
172, 175
dryness, 154–155, 156
lubrication, 154, 156, 171
Vascular invasive cancer, 73, 147
Vegetarian diet, 213
Vinblastine, 259
Vincristine, 259
Visitors. *See also* Family; Friends
breast cancer survivors, 92, 184–185
during hospitalization, 108
Visualization, as therapy, 260
Vitamins
mega-vitamin doses, side-effects, 259
during treatment, 217
vitamin D, 171
vitamin E, 156, 171
Vomiting. *See* Nausea

W

Weight. *See also* Diet; Nutrition; Obesity
as factor in breast cancer, 16, 214
gain, after breast cancer diagnosis,
218
gain, after menopause, 172
gain, during treatment, 172, 175, 176,
216–217
ideal, and management of
lymphedema, 199
maintaining, 214, 217
Wide excision mastectomy. *See* Partial
mastectomy
Will, discussion with family, 243

X

X-rays, chest, 82

Y

Yeast infection, 154

Z

Zofran, 153
Zoladex, 166, 175